How I Quit Drinking (and how you can too)

By

Jackie Elliott

Cover Photography by

Jessica Breeze Photography

Published by Writer Unblocked Publishing

ISBN 978-0-9939542-4-5

Don’t forget to grab your FREE ebook “Ten Simple Step. Get Unstuck & Kick the Booze”

Details at the back!

Contents

Introduction

A while ago I wrote a book called "Sober Ever After". It is a book about me, my relationship with booze, how it started, how booze and I got intimately acquainted, how I used and abused booze and finally, how our relationship became corrosive and destructive. And then, thankfully, ended.

The book was difficult to write.

Anyone who has experienced any form of addiction will know the hardest (well, one of the hardest) aspects to 'recovery', is shining a light on those humiliating, cringe-inducing moments of your life you would most like to forget.

It is, however, one of the most important processes to go through, if you want to be sober (or clean) for the rest of your days.

I was lucky. I do not have a salacious "dead drunk in a ditch on a dark night" kind of story. Again, *lucky*. I have seen, firsthand, the accelerated slide into the abyss, if one is not able to burst through the bubble of denial.

It's not pretty, the abyss. It's full of DUIs, bankruptcy, broken marriages and broken hearts.

I am forever grateful that I only peered over the edge.

I wrote "Sober Ever After" as a warning. To myself mainly, but also to others, who may have heard the tiny but urgent voice saying…" Er, is this normal?"

The answer should come firmly…" No, it is *not*"
That was the message of "Sober Ever After".

"How to Quit Drinking and Live Sober Ever After" is the answer to the question that comes next:

"What do I do now?"

How can I make sobriety stick?

This was the question I asked myself over and over, along with *"why do I keep failing?"*

I had done difficult things before.

I had, in the past, stuck to diets and exercise regimes. I had even trained for several marathons.

So why did I find it so fucking hard to "control" my alcohol intake?

The answer, I found, was a combination of factors.

I wanted to be sober, but I didn't really want to quit drinking.

I wanted to be sober, but I wanted no one to know I was sober.

I wanted to be sober, but I didn't want my life to change.

I discovered that many other people felt the same way. I got an email from a lady, just after she read my first book, saying

"I wish I could just wake up in the morning and not want to drink anymore."

Sober Paths.

At the end of "Sober Ever After" I said this

"I wish I could write a definitive How–To Guide for Quitting Booze. But what worked for me, might not work for you. In sober circles, it's common to hear the phrase "There is no One Size Fits all approach to sobriety"

And that's true, to a certain extent.

But the more relevant question, I think is this:

"How do I get sober and then ***want to stay sober****?"*

So this book aims to answer this question in the following way.

Why is this so hard?

Quitting drinking is hard because of all the bullshit about alcoholism and sobriety we accept.

Hands up who has done any "questionnaires" about drinking habits?

Hands up who has googled "Am I an alcoholic?"

Hands up who has imagined "recovery" as sitting on a hard chair in a circle with homeless people in a Church Hall, drinking bad coffee?

Hands up who can see yourself sitting in the corner, drinking diet coke at a party, while people whisper about you?

My hand is up for all four.

This is how I imagined "alcoholism", "recovery" and "sobriety"

The over-riding aim of this book is to de-bunk *all of this bullshit.*

The Nuts and Bolts of Surviving Sobriety.

The "how-to" part of getting sober is a largely personal choice. I completely agree that there isn't a single approach that works for everyone.

The "Nuts and Bolts" part of this book provides basic strategies and is useful even if you are in a Twelve-Step program and/or attending some kind of group recovery.

While some strategies will work better than others, you still need strategies.

While some of you will keep your "problem" a secret, and others will be open to curious questions, at some point, everyone will face that dilemma and need to make that decision.

As with all "how-to" guides, the best way to use this section, is to "cherry pick".

Living Sober

Living a sober life forever, is a lot different from getting sober.

In sober circles, it's normal to hear sobriety described as a journey or a path (I do this myself), but at some point, you've got to wonder, does this journey end? When can I stop thinking about booze?

I don't think about sobriety as a journey OR a destination any more.

I think about sobriety as a lesson, or a tool that shapes the rest of my life.

Who will benefit from this book?

Anyone who wants to quit drinking, anyone willing to put in some effort, and knows reading about quitting drinking is not the same as doing something about it.

It's for you if you have an open mind, and will try viewing sobriety as a gift for embracing, rather than a life of deprivation.

It's for you, if you can learn from your past, rather than live in your past.

It's not for you if you require medical intervention to help you quit, or if you even suspect you may need medical help. Don't take the risk.

Important Note

You must consult a doctor or a health professional before you attempt to quit drinking if you have any concern about the extent of your physical dependence on booze. Anything you read here is NOT a substitute for proper medical care.

Alcohol dependence is SERIOUS, and stopping abruptly can put your health at risk.

I can't emphasize that enough.

Part One.

A Different "Model" of Sobriety & Laying the Foundation.

"Light tomorrow with today"

Elizabeth Barrett Browning.

Chapter 1.

Finding Answers.

I struggled with booze for years.

In my twenties, I had my booze consumption under strict control. I worked very hard at monitoring my intake, *unless I was stressed.*

It was although my daily "control" was a valve I was constantly tightening, just a little more, and then, when it blew, *it really blew.*

For the last decade before I quit, my drinking was categorized as *extremely risky.*

In my heart I knew this, and occasionally, I would acknowledge out loud that I should "cut down".

But this was much harder than I had expected.

Moderation.

I believe moderation is possible for some people.

In fact, there is research* that supports the notion that some people can effectively 'reset' their relationship with booze.

I attempted to "moderate" many times and failed.

I set myself "rules" for drinking.

For example, one rule was that I would not drink on weekdays. I would only drink at weekends. Except that I always included Frida as "the weekend". And if there happened to be a statutory holiday, well, my "drinking days" extended again.

All my self-imposed rules worked in the beginning, yet disintegrated as time went by.

Not that I was weak.

I was resentful.

Every day I didn't drink, was a day I was depriving myself. Eventually I became angry and resentful about these rules that weren't fair.

My failure to moderate was inevitable.

I believe moderation can be successful, depending on your *mindset* and the role alcohol plays in your life.

I've chatted with many people who largely believe alcohol has almost no role to play in their life at all, but who still want the ability to have the occasional glass of wine with friends, and to accept a glass of champagne at a wedding without making a fuss or pretending to drink it.

I get that.

They are the same people who use those pretty bottle- stoppers in half-finished bottles of wine.

I was never one of those people.

Alcohol played a much more significant role in my life, and control was out of the question. I needed to believe alcohol adds no value to my life whatsoever.

And then, the question is not so much "is moderation possible?" than "why bother?"

Sober Challenges.

In the same way that moderation did not work, Sober Challenges did not change my dysfunctional drinking habits in the long term.

Here's the two main reasons Sober Challenges didn't work for me

First, I didn't want to quit forever. I believed I could 'reset'. Like lots of people I believed a sober challenge would "give my liver a rest" (not a "thing") or *prove to myself that I could quit when I wanted to.*

Just recently, I saw a post on my social media news feed.

"WOO-HOO! I made it through Dry July! And now I'm drinking WINE AGAIN!! Dear Wine, I've MISSED YOU SO MUCH!!!"

After my one and only enforced month of sobriety, I hit the booze again with gusto, convincing myself that I had "detoxed" my system, and had all the evidence I needed, that my drinking wasn't a problem, because I could stop. Whenever I wanted.

Second, I didn't pay attention.

If you are finding it hard to stop drinking a beverage for thirty days, wouldn't that be a red flag? A sign that maybe you have a teensy problem?

It should be, but in my case, I was too busy gritting my teeth through the challenge, crossing off each day on the calendar, rather than focusing on any meaningful insight into my dependence on booze.

Most of us can stop doing / start doing something for thirty days. But if the "something" is to be a permanent lifestyle change, then we need to buy in to it, totally and completely. We need to fall in love with the "something", do it as naturally as breathing, and be horrified at the thought of our life going back to the days when we did/didn't do the "something".

Sobriety, (the "something") cannot be maintained by willpower alone. Even if willpower holds out for a long time, it will always be fragile.

Ever heard a story about someone who was sober for twenty years, then had one drink and fell off the wagon and slipped back into a life of alcohol dependency?

For people who live a life of deprivation, believing they are always missing out, who define themselves by their addiction, relapse simmers just under the surface.

The Disease Model

Is alcoholism a disease? And if so, do I have it?

I researched this question with simultaneous trepidation and hopefulness.

Trepidation I would be forever an outcast, and hopefulness, that somehow this whole sorry situation was not my fault.

I couldn't find a definitive answer.

For every piece of 'research' suggesting that that some of us are genetically pre-disposed to becoming addicted to booze (or anything else), there is a counter-study, with another plausible explanation.

The question consumed me why was I struggling with my drinking?

I found the "elevator theory" of alcohol dependence.

At the top floor, are people who can wander on and off the alcohol elevator at will. These are those people who occasionally have a glass of wine at dinner. Who often go months without drinking an alcoholic beverage because it never crosses their mind.

They might display bewildering behaviour, such as leaving a glass of wine untouched after a few sips, or having an open bottle of white wine in the fridge for so long they have to throw it away.

It's fair to say I was never on the top floors (or only briefly).

Further on down, are the floors for the weekend and holiday binge drinkers. Who would never dream of drinking on a "school night" but are happy to let rip and drink until they vomit over the weekend.

And then you have your "maintenance drinkers". People who drink regularly, almost every day. Never drinking enough to fall over, but over time, experience physical symptoms such as blackouts and erratic behaviour. (I fell into this category).

Further on down, getting near the bottom, are people who have become severely physically dependent on alcohol. Who need medical intervention such as rehab, or hospitalization to detox, and supervision through the first weeks or months of recovery.

It's a broad spectrum, and all drinkers fit on somewhere on the elevator ride. And some people stay on the elevator for the full downwards experience.

Then my question became something different. How do I get off the elevator?

Twelve-Step Programs.

Mention "alcoholism" and the next thought, or at least a few short thoughts afterwards, comes "Alcoholics Anonymous"

Started way back in the 1930s by Bill Wilson, this free organisation has helped countless people shake off their alcohol dependency and become a lifelong "friend of Bill".

They root core beliefs and values in the famous "Twelve-Step Program", addicts helping addicts, and anonymity.

But I didn't want to go to meetings.

Most of what I "knew" about AA was not from direct experience, and I am not critical of AA.

When I first admitted to myself that my tendency to have one too many, was a far bigger problem, I was first filled with dread I would have to stand up in front of a room of strangers and announce

"My name's Jackie and I'm an alcoholic".

The reason I didn't go to start off with, was fear.

The reasons now, are different.

Labels and Language.

Language is powerful. It helps forms our thoughts, beliefs and values.

I do not identify myself as an Alcoholic. I use the term for convenience (for others), but I've found that there are so many misconceptions around the label, that it has become virtually meaningless.

I do not identify myself as "in recovery".

Overall, I believe labels are strictly for soup cans.

The Process

"Steps" or moving through "steps" implies a linear program, at least that's the visual I get. And I don't feel that my journey is linear.

It feels like I've been going round and round in circles sometimes, - or I've taken a detour to sort an issue out, or I've doubled back occasionally!

I just don't feel like it's a straight line, and I wanted to visualize my progress in a way that made sense to me.

Years ago I studied psychology, and during my studies, I came across Abraham Maslow.

Abraham Maslow created Maslow's Hierarchy Of Human Needs.

Picture a pyramid. At the base of the pyramid of needs, is all the stuff we need for basic survival. Food, water, shelter…without this stuff, we need nothing else. Then once these needs are met, we look around for security; we need to feel safe. Moving up the pyramid, we come to love and belonging–our human need to feel accepted into some kind of group. Then, once we feel part of something, we can satisfy our need to elevate our self- esteem, to feel good about ourselves. ONLY then can we fulfil our need (according to Maslow) for self- actualization, basically to fulfil what we perceive as our purpose in life. Achieving our highest human potential. Much later, after completing this pyramid, Maslow added the pinnacle to human needs–transcendence–our spirituality, our altruism.

Despite its simplicity, (humans are complicated creatures after all), the pyramid concept appeals. I like the idea of mastering each stage before climbing the pyramid. So I applied the principle to my own sober journey.

The Hierarchy of Sobriety.

Stage 1–The Basics.

At the bottom of the pyramid are all the skills we need to master for our sober survival–overcoming our fears and denial, the sober strategies we need to use, all the sober tools at our disposal–just about everything we've covered so far.

Stage 2–First Challenges.

As we climb up the pyramid, we need to feel safe and secure and belong. We need our friends and family to accept our new found sobriety. We deal with our fears of stigma, of embarrassment, we face the challenges of being a non- drinker in a boozy world.

Stage 3–Self Esteem.

As we come more comfortable with our sober selves–often the ghost of our boozy past will pop up when we least expect it. We need to come to peace with behaviour we might not be proud of during our drinking days. Maybe, our need to apologise, or reconnect with people who we have alienated.

Stage 4 - Living and Loving Life.

At the top of the pyramid for me is transcendence of sobriety. Here, we are living our lives, not in "recovery", not defined as that person who was a drinker, but as a non- drinker living the best life possible, encompassing all parts of our life–the material, the physical, the intellectual and spiritual.

Self–Awareness & Honesty.

"The truth will set your free, but first it will piss you off." Gloria Steinem.

Whatever path to sobriety you take, self-awareness and honesty are the keys to success.

My drinking years were filled with denial and lies, mostly to myself. The thing is, on some level, I knew the truth. I was caught in this awkward space (cognitive dissonance) of being *uncomfortable in my skin. Like a thief who is always worried about being caught.*

Once I faced the truth about my drinking and behaviour, it was difficult at first to let go of my ego, but the resulting freedom and *relief* was worth it.

References.

'A Theory of Human Motivation" Abraham Maslow, 1943.

Chapter 2

Why Quit?

The foundation of Hierarchy of Sobriety, the solid base you will build on depends on getting one basic truth in place

Why do you want to quit?

As you have picked up this book, I'm assuming that you already have ideas about why you want to quit drinking. It may not be fully defined in your mind. It might just be a vague sense that all is not well, and you have an inkling that your impending sense of doom has something to do with the overflowing garbage bin of empty beer cans and wine bottles.

When I first thought about quitting, on some logical level I knew I was drinking far too much, and that it was probably (definitely) putting my health at risk. Yet, I always negotiated myself out of that fear, I drank wine, they make wine from grapes, grapes are fruit–seriously, how harmful could wine be?

No, I quit because I was miserable.

I was miserable because I had achieved nothing in my life (I thought)

I was miserable because I felt physically unwell most of the time.

I was miserable because people around me were tiring of my bullshit. Drunk Jackie may have been funny at first, but now she was erratic, mean and tedious.

I was miserable because every time I looked in the mirror; I saw a middle-aged loser, who had failed to live up to her potential.

And although I couldn't blame it all on the booze, before I could turn the ship around, I knew my dysfunctional drinking habits had to be the first to go.

Let's look at some of the most compelling reasons for quitting booze.

Health Reasons

The damage that booze is doing to your health SHOULD be the most logical reason to quit, but for lots of us, it's not.

I'm an above average intelligent person, yet I still convinced myself that my habit *wasn't that bad.*

I'm not alone.

I'm not making excuses here, but ignoring the health risks is easier if you have a constant barrage of "propaganda" from the Alcohol Industry.

Via social media platforms, popular TV shows and spurious, biased scientific "research", the narrative that alcohol is harmless and fun and normal has become the loudest.

Early in 2016, government health officials and scientists pushed back.

Citing recent research that linked even small amounts of alcohol consumption with several cancers, the UK Health Minister said (controversially)

"I would like people to make their choice knowing the issues and do as I do when I reach for my glass of wine and think: 'Do I want my glass of wine or do I want to raise my risk of breast cancer?'. And I take a decision each time I have a glass." (as reported in the Guardian, Feb 2016)

Also in February 2016, Dr. Gregory Taylor, Chief Public Health Officer of Canada, released a report that detailed alarming trends of increased health risks associated with drinking.

He said

"Although handled more like a food in Canada, alcohol is a mind-altering drug and there are health risks associated with drinking. Our low risk drinking guidelines do not mean that alcohol is harmless".

But there is a constant push-back from the Alcohol industry.

Following a study by researcher Jennie Connor, University of Otago, the New Zealand Spirits Industry insisted that the findings, that linked seven cancers directly to drinking (at any level), were "misleading".

So who (and what) are we to believe?

The problem is that the waters are constantly muddied.

And we, good ol' Joe Public is pretty frustrated at all these competing "studies", that we pay little attention to any of them.

Until it serves our purpose.

Elliot Aronson, an eminent social psychologist discussed the theory of *cognitive dissonance* in his book "The Social Animal", as it pertained to smoking.

Cognitive dissonance is that awkward feeling of tension that occurs whenever you attempt to hold two opposing cognitions–ideas, beliefs, behaviour, opinions.

For example, a smoker who really enjoys smoking, may experience cognitive dissonance if he or she should read medical evidence that links smoking to cancer. The smoker then has two options to reduce or eliminate that nasty feeling–either give up smoking (hard) or cast around for another piece of 'evidence' that says maybe smoking isn't so bad, or maybe the links to cancer aren't really proven…

Drinkers do that too.

Faced with health studies that warn of the dire consequences of excessive drinking–it's so much easier (than quitting) to cling on to the sensational headlines on social media that proclaim

"Drinking one glass of wine is equivalent to an hour in the gym!"

"Three glasses of champagne per day will reduce the risk of dementia!"

Even if we know on some logical level that these claims are ridiculous, deep down we take comfort that our drinking might not be *that bad, there must be SOME truth to these 'studies' right?*

ER, wrong.

The other problem is that *we never think it will happen to us.*

We believe we will be the exception to the rule. The outlier.

I call this the "Keith Richard's Syndrome."

Now, Keith Richards, (bless him) is a rock icon and is famous for not only surviving but THRIVING against all odds–decades of alcohol, drug and nicotine abuse. It's a compelling narrative, living the rock-and-roll lifestyle, with all its excesses and outliving just about everyone to tell the tale.

And I happen to have a bit of a thing for him, (please don't email me)

But the narrative about Keith Richards–seemingly the picture of health after years of drug and alcohol abuse (or similar) is what your average alcohol-dependent person will hang their hat on. Doesn't have to be Keith Richards per se , but it's amazing to me that so many of my alcohol dependent acquaintances have uncles or aunts who lived to 103, only existing on a bottle of wine a day, and a pound of lard.

Now it seems ridiculous–but this argument for lots of people can be persuasive (plus the whole idea of the rock-and-roll lifestyle).

Now I wonder if you have heard the sentiment - or seen the meme–about a person screeching at full speed into their grave, having lived their life at full throttle, drinking hard, and playing hard?

EVERYONE agrees that we all should live life to the full, but the reality is alcohol abuse will lead to liver failure. The end of a person's life may be in a wheelchair, with weekly visits to the hospital to drain fluid from their body because organs have shut down. This is not rock-and-roll, yet people cling to this "Keith Richard's" illusion.

Often, we don't accept our mortality, or recognize our own part in hastening our demise, until it's too late.

If you (like me) consumed (or are consuming) over the recommended limits of alcohol per week, and/or are regularly getting drunk, then expect damage to your health.

My 'scare' came in the form of blackouts.

Many mornings I would have no recollection of conversations, TV shows, or even getting to bed the night before. And the most frightening aspect was that it was happening frequently, and with less alcohol.

Productivity & Cold Hard Cash.

Hands up! Have you ever slunk into work on a Monday morning, sipping on a water bottle, your stomach doing flip-flops and your head pounding?

(My hand is up).

When you feel like shit, you are not producing your best work. Fact.

Not even you creative types. Before you go all Ernest Hemingway on me, I will take your literary alcohol dependent genius and counter it with one of my own.

Raymond Carver said 'Any artist who is an alcoholic, is an artist despite their alcoholism, not because of it"

This is true.

Imagine if we multiplied all these hours of non-productivity due to alcohol for all employees or business people throughout a whole economy, what would be the cost?

Well, we don't have to imagine, because someone has already done this study, in Australia.

A study by the Australian Education and Rehabilitation Foundation, in 2010, found that the mis- use of alcohol cost the economy approximately $36 BILLION per year, in either actual direct costs to productivity and households, and the more intangible costs to quality of life.

That's a lot of dough.

But if it does not concern you about the economy, what about your own bank account?

Let's use of real-life example. Me.

When I was drinking, I put away about a bottle of wine per day. Let's assume, on the average, I spent $15 per bottle.

7 x 15 = 105

52 (weeks) x 105 = 5460

That's five thousand four hundred and sixty dollars I could have used to reduce debt, to put towards a new car, to spend on a wonderful holiday.

Instead, I spent that money on getting my buzz on, sitting on the couch daily.

AND, this negatively impacted my ability to contribute to the economy in any meaningful way.

A double whammy, hurting my bank balance AND Canada's economy all in one shot. (Or multiple glasses).

And what about the damage to your career?

Some of you may not feel any loyalty to your employer and maybe you hate your job. Maybe the only way you feel you can get through the week is by drowning out your boredom and despair with the booze, *you think*.

But you are also drowning out any ability or motivation to change your life and seriously compromising your future financial freedom.

Your Dreams, Aspirations and Goals.

In the 1970s, my favourite TV show was "The Good Life".

For those of you who did not have access to the BBC, or are not as old as I am (and probably don't remember the "Really Hot Summer of 1976", the Queen's Silver Jubilee) this sitcom was about a couple who decide to become self-sustaining, and live off the grid. Except that they did this in one of the posh suburbs of London, much to the horror of their upper-middle class neighbours. The comedy was the interaction between the neighbours, as the first pig was introduced to the back garden, and they plough the front lawn up for the potato patch, and so on.

I thought it was cool. That you could actually DO that. (I hadn't clued in that it was a *sitcom).* And it was always my dream (and I have pursued it in many ways over the years) to live a life that is *far more simple.*

I love technology, and advances in science, and new inventions. In fact, my husband is an inventor.

I have just always wanted to do two things; grow my food and write my own books.

But life gets remarkably complicated. Before you even realize it.

First, parents, once they have invested into your education have loftier ambitions for you, than weeding the garden daily.

Second, you are told that happiness won't come from the short stories you have lovingly crafted, or carrots.

Third, you need actual money to live on, which doesn't come from the short stories you have lovingly crafted, or carrots.

Fourth, you often meet other people who tell you that accounting is far more exciting than it sounds (it isn't. Not for me anyway) and persuade you to leave the short stories and carrots in a drawer. (metaphor – no carrots were actually left in drawers)

So I abandoned the dreams of my seven-year-old self, and became an accountant, and married a perfectly nice man, and both those things didn't last.

After many years of lots of other things and people not lasting in my life, and a growing realization that time on this planet is short, and I had already mis-used a fair proportion of my allocation-I drank. Because then I wouldn't have to think about it. And handily for me, for once I seemed in sync with lots of other people who had also abandoned the dreams of their seven-year-old selves, and had maybe divorced, or were weighed down with debt and jobs they didn't like, and had similarly become all disillusioned–because they were drinking as well.

So, for a while, it all appeared this would be the way it was *supposed* to be.

Except that it wasn't. And it isn't.

A while ago, I found the first episode of The Good Life on YouTube.

In it, a forty-year-old Tom Goode says…." I haven't got IT right"

"What's "It"?" his wife asks……" I don't know", he answers…

IT.

What we are all looking for. The answer and purpose to our lives.

I know now that "IT" isn't found at the bottom of a wine bottle.

More likely, is that your seven-year-old self already knew what "IT" was.

Mine did.

And after I put down the bottle, and quit the job (er, it really quit me), ploughed up the front garden and wrote stuff again, I found out I will probably never be rich, because money doesn't come from short stories and carrots–but you know what? My happiness DOES come from those dreams and aspirations.

If you, like me, are bored, disillusioned or just plain unhappy with your life, alcohol will work to numb that feeling. In the short term.

In the long term, alcohol will add to your anxiety, your fears that life is just passing you by (it is), and booze will just compound your unhappiness.

Although I cannot guarantee that you will achieve the dreams of your seven-year-old self, merely by quitting the booze (especially if you wanted to be a ballerina), I can guarantee that your chances for a meaningful change in your life, for *happiness* are very much increased.

It was fun and now it's not

When we boil it down to the essential elements, the main reason why people should quit drinking (and why I did) is that drinking USED to be fun….but now it's not.

Most of us start drinking in our teens (even if it's illegal). We do it to rebel, to push boundaries, we react to peer pressure; we are curious…..all of this is normal. For most of us.

Others start because there is a family history of drinking, and therefore it seems like the normal thing to do.

Whatever the reason for starting, no one ever intends to end up with a drinking problem.

That usually creeps up on us, stealthily.

Looking back, I remember many fun times when I was tipsy….. a whole gaggle of us, holding hands, laughing and singing off-key to Dexy's Midnight Runners…. I remember feeling the warmth and joy as I chinked glasses of champagne when I first got engaged, romantic sips of wine on a trip to Italy. I wouldn't change any of these experiences for the world.

But gradually, the regular intoxication turned me mean, instead of carefree.

I became rude, boorish, unpredictable.

I writhed in humiliation at 3.00am in the morning.

I became an embarrassment to my husband, who tried at first to laugh it off, but finally lost patience enough, that he stopped accepting invitations on our behalf, preferring to watch me pass out on the couch, rather than risk a drunken scene.

It wasn't fun to drink anymore.

It wasn't fun for me.

It wasn't fun for anyone.

The Change in Drinking.

The change in my drinking came the day I uttered the words

"I really need a drink".

Drinking stopped being a "nice to have" and turned into a "need to have".

I stopped enjoying alcohol, and I started using alcohol.

It was a fundamental shift in my mindset towards booze and I didn't even notice.

One reason I didn't feel the change, was maybe because all the cues I was getting from society, media and social platforms…. were that this *need* for alcohol was not only normal, it was totally, well, cool.

Cool parents, cool businesswomen, sophisticated women everywhere relied on booze to be their "liquid helper" for life.

Ann Dowsett Johnston, in her memoir "Drink" and also in her TEDtalk says women's dysfunction drinking is influenced by three factors–childhood trauma, the availability of booze and…… *marketing.*

After the Women's Liberation movement in the 1970s, when women were earning disposable incomes of their own–Dowsett Johnston argues that the Alcohol Industry identified women as a "marketing segment" that was "under-performing", and henceforth, they did something about it.

It makes sense.

When I think back to the 1990s, it was the rise of the 'ladette' culture in the UK. Women were frequenting bars and nightclubs, having "Girl's Night Out" and it became the new badge of feminism to be drinking the boys under the table.

It was the "Sex in the City" era–women were openly boozing during the day, and simultaneously, in the stores, wines were popping up with names like "Mummy Juice", "Bitch" and "Therapy".

Fast forward a decade or so, and wine in particular has become our 'go to' stress reliever.

Whereas my mum would get into work and pop the kettle on, it's normal now, to uncork and unwind with a glass of something chilled.

Look at it this way. The Alcohol industry won't get rich if we confine our drinking to the odd glass of wine at dinner, or social events. No, the real money is from regular (every day) purchases.

Instead of traditional direct advertising–there are few "in your face" ads that tell you to drink more–the industry relies on the more insidious social media platforms, portrayal of elegant women in TV shows, and the relentless message we NEED the booze to survive our hectic, stressful lives.

And it works.

Your Reasons For Quitting.

Why do YOU want to quit drinking?

There are many great reasons to quit–health, wealth and happiness to name three, but unless you can identify your *specific* reasons, the quitting won't stick.

How often have you been on a diet, or started an exercise regime, only to abandon it or "cheat" within the first few days? How many times have you started off, really motivated and fired up….only to talk yourself out of it when you don't achieve instant results?

The entire Diet Industry relies on the fact we have very little willpower.

Quitting drinking is the same.

"White knuckling" it will only work for a limited time.

The most effective way to quit drinking is to *want* to quit rather than think you *should* quit.

The first step in quitting drinking is to identify all the reasons you WANT to put down the bottle.

When sobriety really 'stuck' for me, I made two lists. The first was all the things I hated about drinking.

The second was all the things I wanted to improve in my life I believed stopping drinking could help me achieve.

Your first step is to spend a few minutes writing your own lists.

References

Aronson, Elliott, The Social Animal, W.H Freeman & Co, 1995 Seventh Ed, Chapter 5 Self Justification.

Dowsett Johnston, Ann, Drink, Harper Perennial, 2014.

Chapter 3

Facing Fear

Once you have figured out all those reasons for quitting, you may ask yourself this:

Why on earth didn't I quit drinking earlier? Why did I allow myself to be miserable for all those years?

Although I knew I was unhappy and unwell, I always seemed to resist change.

The reason was simple.

I was afraid.

Fear has different names.

Procrastination.

Worry.

Laziness.

It was always easier to think to myself, "I'll quit on Monday". And then when Monday came, there was always another excuse.

FEAR is often the reason it takes so long for people to quit drinking.

What Are We Fearful About?

The fear of quitting often outweighs the fear of NOT quitting.

It's also easier to find people to assuage fears about NOT quitting–usually because fear also traps them in a cycle–and who wants to be frightened alone?

Your own fears, and those of the surrounding people, form this "bubble" that is hard to escape.

The thing about FEAR, is that it is part of life. You can never fully escape from it. BUT, you can learn to live with it.

Confound FEAR with LOGIC.

Fear hates logic.

Because FEAR is illogical.

Most of the things that frighten us *haven't happened.*

I base most of our fears on "what if" scenarios in our head.

What if my husband doesn't love me if I quit drinking?

What if I get left out of parties if I'm sober?

If we pepper our FEAR with the logical arguments…

"Surely our marriage is based on more than a beverage. Surely my husband loves me enough to care about my health. How about I have a conversation with him and find out what he thinks?"

…..we often find that none of our fears are real.

Logic is Fear's kryptonite.

FEAR really hates ACTION.

I really wish I had a dollar for everyone who has said or emailed

"It wasn't anywhere near as bad as I thought it would be!"

Think about the last time you did something you were nervous about–zip lining, ski-ing, an interview, socializing without a drink in your hand…….. didn't the fear completely disappear the minute you were *actually doing what you were nervous about?*

I remember the build-up to exams. The sweaty palms, butterflies in my stomach, but the minute I started scribbling, all the fear evaporated.

It's the same when you quit drinking. The minute you face a hurdle–a celebration, Christmas, or a wedding–the fear diminishes and confidence takes its place.

The way to escape is to DO rather than THINK

FEAR doesn't EXIST in the PRESENT.

Every action, every decision, even the words we utter *today will have an effect, good or bad, on our future.*

The way to confront our fears, is to focus on the present.

Worried about that dinner party next Saturday?

Focus on not drinking today, and all the positive benefits of being sober now. Building your confidence today, will positively affect the outcome on Saturday.

When I start "catastrophizing" about our financial future; what if we sell nothing this week? How will we pay our bills? How long before we are living under a bridge?–I take a deep breath and focus on the piece of paper, or the email in front of me.

Because I know if all my mental bandwidth is full of "what ifs", I won't be sending emails to clients, or talking to suppliers, or doing all the hundred tasks that WILL bring us sales.

FEAR can be a self-fulling prophecy if you let it. So focus on *what you can do right now,* and let your positive actions and decision decide your future.

So let's examine some common fears and blast them with our new three-point plan, Logic, Action and staying in the present.

"I'm Afraid that I'm an Alcoholic"

This is a really common fear. We picture ourselves drunkenly staggering around in our dirty housecoat, screaming obscenities at the kids, and spending our savings on cheap cider, until finally we are alone, abandoned by our loved ones.....

There are people whose lives are ruined by addiction to alcohol and drugs. Who end up losing jobs and houses, marriages and children.

But this is not the inevitable path that dysfunctional drinkers follow.

When I first knew booze, might, just might, be an issue, I dismissed that thought, repeatedly.

Silly right? How could I possibly be an alcoholic? As far as I was aware, no one in my family had a drinking problem. So it couldn't be in my genes right? Unless I had some genetic mutation....... but although I got drunk "occasionally", it wasn't really affecting my life.... I hadn't got a DUI (yet) or a (another) divorce? And I was still working.....

I based all my assumptions about my drinking on a stereotype of an alcoholic I carried around with me.

I wasn't an alcoholic *until it got that bad. Until I reached some symbolic "rock bottom".*

But instead of being a warning–*maybe I had better stop now, before it gets too late*–bizarrely, I attempted to *drink my way through the problem.*

In my twisted logic, I assumed that BECAUSE I was worried about being an alcoholic, I COULDN'T POSSIBLY BE an alcoholic, because everyone knows REAL alcoholics are in complete denial. So, in order to "prove" to myself that I was "fine", I shouldn't STOP drinking, I should carry on, and not give it another thought.

This kind of perverted reasoning, I've found, is also common.

The FEAR of being an alcoholic, instead of curtailing consumption–actually does the reverse.

So let's dispel some myths.

There is no ONE definition of Alcoholism

If you ask a dozen scientists, addiction counsellors, doctors and drunks to describe exactly what alcoholism is, you'll get two dozen explanations.

Is it a disease? Is it hereditary? Is it dependent on how much I drink? Or how often? Or if I get drunk?

If you have spent hours fretting over those online questionnaires, as I did, it may strike you how many subjective questions there are.

For example, a question such as "has your drinking ever affected your job?" is a hard one to answer. Have I ever got fired because I was drinking? No. But I certainly phoned in sick more than once with the Mysterious Monday "flu" and spent the day under the duvet sleeping off the excesses of the weekend...

My "aha" moment around this fear came about a year after I had quit. I was still a little sensitive around the whole notion of being "sober" and the connotations it implied, but I was delighted to answer, when asked by my doctor, how much alcohol I consumed in a week–that I drank ZERO booze now!

After a brief discussion about why I had quit, which involved no detailed analysis of how many units I was consuming, or any adverse physical symptoms I had experienced, my doctor cheerfully said,

"I'll mark you down as a dry alcoholic on your file"

It flabbergasted me.

And I realized then that the whole concept of "alcoholism" was complete bullshit.

I don't know what alcoholism is. And my doctor doesn't appear to either.

So it makes NO LOGICAL SENSE to wear a label which I, and many other people don't understand or can define.

One thing I know for sure, is that alcoholism doesn't exist without.... alcohol.

If you are fearful of BEING an alcoholic, or descending into the abyss of alcoholism, the action of putting down the bottle will quash that fear right away.

"I'm Afraid That It Will Be Too Hard to Quit"

I can answer that one right away.

Yes. It WILL be hard, and you'll wonder why you bothered. You'll look on enviously as other people crack open a "cold one" or swill a full-bodied red around in their glass, or sip on an oaky single malt... and you'll think, "Fuck it. This is too hard"

But if you work through the hard bits, even if they make you *literally cry actual tears* you'll be rewarded by crystal clear mornings, warming your hands on a coffee mug as the sun filters through the trees, moments of pure joy as you are fully present with your children.....or moments of quiet exhilaration and fulfillment as you marvel at your creative accomplishments.

Sobriety has been one of the hardest things I have done. Although it is just a simple *inaction*–just not drinking a particular beverage–the hard parts (and the best parts) are the ongoing lessons in self-awareness.

And you know what? I didn't discover that I was irresponsible, lazy, feckless and worthless, as I had suspected during my drinking days. I turned out to be productive, creative, loving and *worthy*.

I would never have figured that out if I hadn't pushed through all the "hard bits" of sobriety.

What will People Think?

Why do we get so tied up in knots about this? If I knew the answer to this, I would be *really really rich*.

Of course, the simple answer is to say "who cares what people think?" But this bumper sticker answer doesn't cut it for most of us because *we all care what other people think*.

Because we are social beings who want to be accepted, loved and respected, we hang around with those people who at least appear to accept, love and respect us. For who we are, and how we behave.

So if we drink a lot, we hang around with people who drink too–because they will tend to be accepting–even encouraging that behaviour and lifestyle.

We gravitate towards "our people".

So once we make a fundamental change to our lifestyle, it stands to reason that some of "our people" will be a little unsettled, and not altogether supportive of our new choices.

I used to be part of a group of women who got together regularly to drink. We dressed it up as "cooking new recipes" or "crafts"–but basically we met in the afternoons, cracked open the wine and drank until we were too drunk to care about the meal or the holiday crafts.

After a while, the group of women got a little smaller, as some ladies (understandably) didn't find these drunken afternoons fun at all, and drifted away….until there were only the 'hard core" drinkers, those of us who were there for the wine.

I see none of these women any more.

None of them were openly hostile about my sobriety, but none of them were particularly supportive either.

I figured out later, or course, that the connectivity of this group completely revolved around the wine. Not conversation, activities, shared interests or values, but the booze in my glass.

It occurred to me that since I wasn't drinking, and no longer attended these boozy afternoons–they probably didn't think "badly" of me, *they more likely didn't think about me at all…*

We will talk at length about finding a new tribe, later in the book, but suffice to say, that although I no longer see my "Afternoon Boozy Ladies", I still have many friends, and our connections go deeper than just the beverage I drink.

What Will Life Be Like Without Booze?

This is the Big One.

Our biggest fear is change. Of losing our comfort zone, the reassuring familiarity of our life. The fear of feeling like the new girl in class, all awkward and lonely.

The sad fact is that many of us settle for a life that doesn't make us happy just because the FEAR of changing it, is so overwhelming.

But here's the problem with that thinking; *Life changes anyway.*

Take a moment to look back over your life. I bet there have been huge changes you didn't plan for, or didn't want. But they happened anyway.

Death, divorce, sickness–these are the harder trials we have to bear. But sometimes JOYOUS changes get thrust upon us too–births, relationships, friendships, travel, careers–all changes we may not have sought out, but fell into our laps, with laughter and hugs.

Not ALL change is bad.

Much of our fear of life without booze, has been constructed by other people. People, who have a vested interest in our continuing drinking.

People, who want you to believe celebrations are bland without the champagne, or the BBQ is DULL without the beer and more troubling, that parenthood is impossibly hard without wine, or that even sports and fitness need to be pepped up with a little "after–workout" drinky.

Those people see you as a creator of profits. A consumer. Data on a chart. Figures in a sales report.

The fact is that MOST people don't drink, or drink very little.

None of that is clear to us while we are drinking. We seek "evidence" to support our own behaviour, and the story that the Alcohol Industry wants us to believe. We stay in our bubble, invested in our thinking whatever the occasion…

"there's a wine for that…."

One of my most shocking "discoveries" when I put down my wineglass and looked around…… *hardly anyone had been drinking all of this time.*

Not all of us drink to be part of the cool crowd.

Some of us drink to hide or escape from something in our life. It could be a trauma or tragedy, or it could be the quiet desperation of a relationship that's not working out, or financial worries, or.. or….

You don't need me to tell you that a bottle of wine will solve nothing.

When I quit and the fog lifted, I surveyed the wreckage.

Luckily for me, my marriage was still intact. But my finances and career were not.

I won't sugar-coat it, whatever you have been putting off facing, probably hasn't gone away. Probably, sticking your head in the sand (booze) hasn't helped at all. And probably, it will be a whole lot harder to deal with NOW, than if you had figured it out a long time ago.

That's the bad news.

The good news is that this sober journey will equip you with new skills and coping mechanisms. With a new clarity of thought and purpose. Most importantly, with the ability to recognise when you need help and the resources to find it.

Far from being a life that is deprived and wanting, a sober life can be anything you want it to be; full of opportunity and excitement.

I feared sobriety because I thought it was the destination.

I didn't realise that sobriety was just the start.

Get your fears out in the open. Make a note of all the worries you have RIGHT NOW about quitting drinking. As you read through this book, note down any ACTIONS you can take to dispel these fears.

Summary of Part 1

- "Cutting down" or "moderation" does not work for many people
- "Sober Challenges" may not be successful because they do not help you "reset" drinking habits, and do not address the underlying reasons for dysfunctional drinking.
- There are many competing theories for the reasons for drinking problems, and trying to find a definitive answer can be confusing and all-consuming (and not helpful)
- The 'Elevator Theory" is a model that not only explains the progression of dysfunctional drinking, but also offers hope for reversal.
- Twelve Step Programs and the language used, may not resonate with everyone.
- A more helpful approach follows a Sobriety Pyramid structure – building on progress. This book is based on that model.
- Self-awareness and truthfulness underpin success.
- Understanding your "why" forms the base of your Sobriety Pyramid.

- Reasons for quitting can include your health, finances, relationships and self-esteem. It's important to identify your reasons at the start.
- FEAR is often a factor in our resistance to quit.
- You may have fears about change, what people think, and your chances of success.
- You cannot conquer fear completely, but you can learn to live with it, by applying logical arguments, focusing on the present, and taking action.

Part Two

The “Nuts & Bolts” of Quitting Drinking.

“We cannot solve our problems with the same thinking we used when we created them”

Albert Einstein

Chapter 4

Getting Started

You've decided that it's time to quit. You've made the decision. You know it's the right one, because you've weighed the pros and cons.

So you're excited to embark on this new sober life right?

No?

Not feeling *ready* yet?

Thinking you might leave it a bit longer? Maybe you have a family wedding to attend, or maybe an all-inclusive holiday in Mexico? Maybe it would be easier to focus on being sober after that celebration/holiday/whatever?

Well, here's the thing.

Of course you're not ready. None of us ever is ready for a big lifestyle change. And that's the problem with readiness–we expend an awful lot of energy on "getting ready" rather than just getting on with it.

Getting ready is really another way of describing procrastination. And procrastination, in these situations is really another version of FEAR.

We are basically afraid of making the change and therefore we keep telling ourselves that we are just waiting until we are ready.

And it is convenient. There are thousands of well-meaning people out there who will tell you comfortingly–don't worry, you'll do this when you are READY….

As if one day, there will be a bolt of lightning, and you'll wake up READY for a sober life. In fact, I get several messages every week from people who tell me something similar…. I wish I could wake up and not want to drink…. which is basically the same as saying… I wish I were READY for a sober life.

That magical day when you are ready? You might as well be waiting for a unicorn sighting.

So buckle up, we will take the plunge together…… three, two, one…… jump!

Taking Action

It's a little weird talking about *action* in relation to sobriety, because the KEY to not drinking is….. er, *not drinking* which is an "inaction".

The BIG SECRET to eliminating booze from your life, is to just stop drinking booze.

It's that simple.

And I know at this point, you may be feeling a little annoyed that I've pointed out the blindingly obvious, and you may be composing an email right now to ask for your money back, BUT there is a point to me irritating you so soon in this book.

It IS simple. (Note I didn't say "easy"). It is NOT complicated. The end goal for you is to live your life without drinking a particular beverage.

That's it.

And I want you to remember this.

Even come back and re-read it if you want every time you get overwhelmed or frustrated or feel like screaming into your pillow, (which I did, on more than one occasion).

The end goal is simple.

Everything else we talk about here are ACTIONS that help you achieve an INACTION.

Planning

When I quit drinking, I didn't have a plan. I did not understand (at the time) that the last time I drank an alcoholic beverage would be on 8th May 2015.

I was helping to cater a wedding. I was attempting to roast a huge side of beef in a tiny oven that refused to warm up. In contrast, I was hot, irritated and perspiring. Outside, my husband was grilling chicken on a BBQ. All around him, people were laughing and enjoying the spring sunshine, and of course, drinking heavily.

Instead of pouring myself a glass of iced water, I grumpily grabbed a can of (warm) beer. I wanted to be drinking and having fun, instead of being stuck in the kitchen.

I watched one lady, dressed in a beautiful black and white dress, lean on the man next to her. She was laughing a little too loudly, and her face was flushed, as she staggered a little and grabbed his arm. She laughed even more hysterically, and as someone else reached out to steady her, she swung her body backwards, lost her footing and plunged towards the BBQ.

My husband grabbed her before she got smothered in the grease. The BBQ remained upright, but the lady, still laughing, was sitting on the ground, her legs splayed outwards like a small child.

I saw myself.

I saw the lady's partner help her to her feet. I saw him wave away the small crowd of people who had been attracted by the commotion. I knew what he was saying.

"Oh, she'll be fine, she just had a bit too much to drink,"

I wondered if her behaviour had embarrassed him as many times as my husband cringed at MY drunken antics.

And I poured away the rest of the warm beer.

I have not had a drink since, and the following plans and actions (the nuts and bolts of quitting) were all instrumental in keeping me sober.

They will help you too.

 # Remove all Alcohol from the Immediate Environment.

This seems obvious right?

But I always get a lot of pushback when I suggest this.

"It seems so *drastic....*"

"My husband still wants to drink"

"But I love to entertain, I have to have wine for visitors,"

Yes, all of these situations are obstacles. And all problems and obstacles have a solution if you are willing to look.

It's not drastic to remove a beverage from your house, if you are never intending to drink it again. What you are saying is this:

"I'm afraid to remove the booze from my house, because it will be proof I have a problem, and I don't want to have a problem. If I remove all the booze, then this situation becomes real. And scary."

You are moving outside your comfort zone. This is new.

"Change is unfamiliar. Change causes incompetence," Seth Godin.

For the first little while, shedding your drinking habit will feel like a lot like being the new girl (or boy) at school. Everything will be unfamiliar, you won't know where to sit, what's next on the timetable or even where to hang your coat. You will feel awkward and vulnerable. You won't have your 'comfort booze blanket' to hang on to.

That's OK.

It's OK to feel 'new'.

Over time, just as you did at school, you'll get used to the new routine and grow in confidence. It won't bother you, in time, to have alcohol in the house. Same as you didn't need or even notice your comfort blanket lying around when you were a kid, because you were too busy getting on with your life– you won't feel the urge to pick up the bottle, every time you see one.

But until then, a half-finished bottle of chardonnay chilling in the fridge will sing to you like Dante's Sirens.

So get rid of it.

 # Speak Your Plan.

On my Day 2, I casually mentioned to my husband…..

"I'm not going to be drinking for a while…"

Now, this "proclamation" did not result in a choir of angels singing the "hallejuhah chorus" or tears of joy from my husband.

Nope, all I got was an eye-roll, because frankly, he had seen this movie before.

It went like this.

9.00am

ME: I've decided to QUIT drinking FOREVER!!

HUSBAND: So I shouldn't buy you wine ever again?

ME: NO! NEVER EVER AGAIN!!

5.00pm

ME: COULD YOU GET ME WINE PLEASE?

HUSBAND: I thought you weren't drinking ever, ever again?

ME: IF YOU LOVED ME YOU WOULD BUY ME WINE RIGHT NOW!!

If this scenario is familiar, then this time, *show* your loved one your new commitment, because like me, you may have a "trust issue" around this.

I suggest that you firstly TELL your significant other, and all the other relevant adults in your household you are not drinking *at the moment (no need to bare your soul),* and once you have removed all the booze from your house (that is yours), then calmly ask them to refrain from purchasing booze for you and if they want to drink, please *find their own space to keep their alcohol.*

My husband continued to drink after I quit, and he still does.

He purchases a bottle of whiskey when he wants to, and he keeps it on the top shelf of the dining room cupboard. As I only ever drank his whiskey once I had polished off all the wine, having the whiskey in the house wasn't a problem.

If other people in your house drink the same beverage as you, then this will be harder. And later on, we'll work through some coping strategies, but right now, try to elicit support, remembering you may (unsurprisingly) face some skepticism at first.

On the other hand, you may get a reaction you weren't expecting.

I thought I had hidden my 'problem" drinking rather well. I was careful about disposing of my recycling. I always made sure that there was the "right" amount of booze in the house, so it never *looked* as if I had been drinking alone.

But I could not hide my erratic behaviour at the end.

I couldn't hide I rarely remembered going to bed, or watching TV shows, or conversations I had in the evenings, after I had started drinking. I didn't recall posting stupid stuff on Facebook, or picking fights with my beleaguered husband.

I couldn't hide my hangovers in the morning anymore, or my wine belly, my flushed skin, and my lack of enthusiasm for…..*well, anything except for wine.*

Although my husband was initially skeptical that I would quit for good, he was also relieved that I was at least trying.

And so I received lots of quiet support.

Hopefully, you will too.

 # Adopt an Alcohol "Policy"

Our house used to be a "party central".

I loved people dropping in because it gave me an excuse to crack open another bottle of wine!

At first, it confused people.

Tea or coffee? I asked "I'm not drinking at the moment, so we don't have wine,"

Here's what happened.

The people who used to drop in for free wine and a party, stopped showing up, pretty quickly.

The people who *actually enjoyed our company continued to visit because they didn't give a shit about the beverage I offered them!*

It was a revelation.

We still entertain, or course.

These days, I remind people that if they would like wine with dinner to please bring their own, otherwise I have lots of non-alcoholic options.

I have only ever had someone get snotty about it once, and now I just don't invite her.

Planning How To Deal With Cravings.

You may not know it until you stop, but drinking consumes much of your time.

As soon as I poured that first glass of wine, the rest of my entire evening was wiped out. Weekends were worse because I started earlier.

Countless times, I would "just reward myself with half a glass" in the middle of doing laundry–and there the clothes would sit, either damp in the washing machine until they started to smell a few days later, or a creased pile that never quite made it to the drawers and closet.

I really came to appreciate this gift of time that sobriety had given me, especially my hangover free mornings, but in the beginning, I really needed SOMETHING to distract me.

As my grandmother always used to say

"The devil makes work for idle hands."

In my case, and maybe yours–it is the Wine Witch that has evil plans for our idleness, so we HAVE to plan distractions to keep her at bay.

The "Wine Witch" is just the persona we give to CRAVINGS.

Cravings–let's look at the actual definition.

"To Crave," is to "long for", "to desire greatly" "to hanker after".

It doesn't mean "if I don't get this now, I will die."

How many times have you seen a small child cry at the supermarket when mum won't buy candy? Maybe you've seen the "toddler meltdown" when the child doesn't get what they want RIGHT NOW. I bet you (as I have done) have been sympathetic to the parent because they are NOT being mean to their kid, they are depriving them of something that is not good for them. This action is not pleasant now, but it will reap great rewards later, when the kid avoids multiple trips to the dentist.

I want you to think of your cravings as "Your Inner Toddler". An unreasonable, shrieking toddler having a tantrum–imagine your toddler bawling, collapsed to the floor, pounding his or her little fists and heels on the ground.

Ridiculous, right?

OK, now we will calm this little dude right down.

1. Distraction.

We've all seen this. Maybe you have done it. Distracting toddlers with other "shiny objects" to get their attention away from the conniption and focused on something else.

As cravings are most likely to be psychological than physical after the first week or so, (all traces of alcohol leave the body within five to ten days of consumption)–the best distractions are those that really occupy the mind.

I'll cover this is more detail in the Sober Toolbox section, but the most beneficial distraction techniques are active rather than passive.

For instance, binge watching Netflix is "passive". You sit and let the entertainment wash over you. It's easy to let your mind wander back to the pesky cravings.

If, however, you are reading, or doing something creative, it requires interaction and focus. You are far less likely to think about drinking.

2. Escape.

Question: When are you more likely to experience an urge to drink?

Answer: When you are faced with other people drinking and alcohol is readily available.

Sometimes the only way to deal with the screaming toddler is to *run away.*

Remove yourself from the situation.

3. Acceptance.

Every toddler has the occasional tantrum. It's normal. They erupt when they want one thing….. *attention.*

Craving are exactly the same. They demand your attention, and because they are uncomfortable, we want them to stop as soon as possible. So we give in.

Like screaming toddlers, if you calmly sit with cravings refusing to give in to their demands, eventually they will stop *all on their own.*

And if you can do this the next time, and the time after that–just as the toddler learns that throwing a screaming fit is not working, your cravings will also subside.

Is it All Just a Bad Habit?

Alcohol dependency is far too complex to treat merely as a bad habit that requires "breaking". There are many interacting factors–physical, psychological and environmental–all intersecting in unique ways for each one of us.

However, some of our drinking behaviour is habitual, and I believe that understanding and identifying those times when we drink "just because" is helpful for the first weeks of sobriety.

I recommend reading the excellent "The Power of Habit" by Charles Duhigg, if you want to delve deep into the psychology of making and breaking habits, but in the meantime, here's a summary.

A "habit" is an action or behaviour we perform without even thinking about it, like automatically pouring a glass of wine when you walk through the door at the end of the workday, without stopping to consider whether you want it.

A habit has three components–a "cue" (or trigger), a routine and a reward. So using the example above, the "trigger" would be getting home after the workday, the routine would be pouring and drinking a glass of wine, and the reward would be the feeling of relaxation, say.

So how do we "break" the habit?

Well, we follow the Golden Rule of Habit Change.

"If you use the same cue and provide the same reward, you can shift the routine and change the habit. Almost any behaviour can be transformed if the cue and the reward stay the same," (Charles Duhigg, The Power of Habit, pg 62).

So, again using our example–our trigger is getting home from work and our reward is relaxation. All we have to do to change our routine. We have to substitute the glass of wine for something else that provides us with the same relaxation.

Breaking That Habit.

Start by identifying your "triggers'.

A trigger in the context of drinking and trying not to drink is an event, situation, person or feeling. It is anything that sets off an urge to drink.

Some common triggers could be;

1. Stress. This is common. Either daily stress, or an ongoing period of stress–or one of those unforeseen life events that smack us round the head (figuratively speaking) can cause the strongest of us to want to reach for the bottle.

2. People. Certain people can drive you to drink. But more likely, social situations, drinking buddies can either knowingly coerce you to drink–or all of that drunken socializing can be a trigger to join in–especially if we can conveniently put out of our minds the inevitable hangover that follows the aforementioned drunken socializing. It may be people online. A certain blogger or social media site.

3. Activities. Certain activities we associate with drinking can be a "trigger". For me, a big trigger was cooking. Standing in the kitchen, chopping away with a glass of wine on the counter. But it could be the book club night, ladies' night at the golf club or any activity you used to do accompanied by booze.

4. Boredom. This is a trigger that maybe we don't really want to acknowledge. It presents us in a better light if we say "Oh I'm so stressed, that's why I drink"…. rather than, I couldn't think of anything else to do, so I just got drunk in front of Netflix.

   But, facing your truth is a big part of this. I'll go first. BOREDOM was a HUGE trigger for me. Being left alone in the house, for a day or two equalled a big 'ol solo wine fest for Jackie.

5. Fake booze. I was a wine drinker, so I've found that non-alcoholic beer was a great help at the beginning, and now I've found a nice one I drink regularly. This may not work for you.

The first thing you need to know about triggers is this:

"All triggers are created equal". And although certain triggers may cause a more powerful urge to drink than others, there are no triggers that are "better" than others, or that give you "special dispensation". And the consequences are exactly the same, namely, a hangover and self- loathing.

Once you have a list of triggers, the next job is to change the routines you associate with those triggers. This is where the Sober Tool Box comes in.

The Sober Tool Box.

A Sober Toolbox is your very own collection of sober strategies, which you lean on like a War Chest. Or, better still, a *Hope Chest.*

The great thing about Sober Toolboxes, is that they are flexible. You can add to them, or discard when necessary.

But there are some basics you can include,

A Non-Alcoholic Beverage to replace the Boozy Beverage

There is much debate around whether it is a good idea to switch to the Non Alcoholic variety of your previous Boozy Beverage. That's a personal decision. Some people find it comforting to have something that looks the same especially in the first weeks because it doesn't draw attention to the fact you are not drinking. But other people find it "triggery". I tried some NA beverages, and I quite liked fake beer, and I still have a few in the fridge. But after the first couple of weeks when I was clinging on to them, I found that soda water was fine.

The thing is to find something you like, to use your best glassware, or fancy cup, or cute teapot, and *treat yourself.*

Sometimes, all you need to beat the cravings, is to take a few moments to make yourself feel special.

A Project.

Or several projects. If there are projects around the house that are half finished, so much the better.

When the Wine Witch comes calling, the most effective thing you can say is…." Go away. I'm busy" *(you can be as forceful as you like)*. And it's helpful if you really *are* busy.

If you have got nothing that needs finishing, then go for the de-cluttering. Re-decorate a room. Create a sanctuary for yourself.

Plant a garden, or window boxes.

I recommend a project that requires physical/manual exertion rather than mental, because it's good to get out of your head, and DO rather than THINK.

So put together a list of projects and drop it into your Sober Toolbox.

De- Stresser Technique.

There will be times you feel panicky or overwhelmed.

That's normal. Don't worry.

But in times like this, you'll need a technique or strategy to calm you down.

You might like to try meditation. If you are new to meditations, you can try a guided meditation.

A Treat!

Feeling left- out? Deprived? Boost yourself with a treat! Yes, it could be Rocky-Road ice cream, with extra chunks of sugary goodness, OR a little healthier option could be a new nail polish. A haircut or anything that 'rewards' you. I 'invested' in a Kindle, and not only did it immediately make me feel good, it was also the self-gift that kept on giving. I once again became an avid reader. And downloading a book and sneaking off to the bedroom for an hour's read also became one of my Sober Tools.

note: Don't feel guilty about sugary treats. It's a common practice to turn to ice cream or candy. But make sure that you include healthy stuff in your diet too. Eventually, the need for sugar will subside.

A Place of Sanctuary

Somewhere you can go when you feel overwhelmed. Or you want to cry in private. I go to my greenhouse, or my garden. I faff about out there until I feel better. It can be anywhere, a favourite walk, your bedroom, a chair in your office with a comfort blanket–somewhere where you feel safe and calm.

A Blog or Journal

It doesn't have to be a public blog (but that can help you connect with other souls in the Sober Cyberverse), it can just be daily scribbles that get all those "mind monkey" thoughts out of your head and onto the page. It can be a therapeutic process. And it's safe. You can whine, be angry, write down your deepest darkest thoughts and get it all out there on the page. (Make sure you hide it, it's not one of those things you want read out at Thanksgiving Dinner…)

A Creative Endeavour

We are born to be creative. We make things with our hands, or create music or stories, or solutions to problems. So often, we believe "creativity" only means "arts and crafts", it's only for "artsy" people, and is really rather frivolous, that you are not "good" at it, or that it should only be an indulgence when all the "important" stuff is finished.

I believed all of the above. So this was a tool I knew I should try, but I was resistant! Until one day, I painted (!) a really terrible picture. And I had *so much fun! And I totally lost myself for a few hours..*

That's the great benefit. When we are being creative–whatever it is–we get into the flow, we are completely focused, we are caught up in the moment. And it is everything we need to lift our spirits and keep the Mind Monkeys or Wine Witch at bay!

So get out your sewing machine, or watercolours, or carving, or music.

Something Soulful

Something that connects you to your Higher Power. Now, some people get 'put off' when they read or hear the phrase "Higher Power".

But this can mean different things to different people. Your Higher Power can mean your God, your Higher Self, your intuition, your Spiritual self. And we can access our own Higher Power by whatever means feel right for us. So prayer works. Meditation works. Oils and Healing Crystals work.

Anything that helps you connect on a spiritual level.

Now, if that seems a little "woo woo" for some people, I get it. But there's something about this sober journey that affects you (in a positive way), that gets you asking questions about all kinds of Big Stuff.

It's important. So when it happens, work with it.

A Sober Tribe

You need a "tribe". People who "get" you, support you, nurture you. It can be a tribe of one person or many people. They can be real life people that meet you for coffee, or they can be online friends, or email buddies. You can find them at meetings, you can find them through blogs, *but you must find them.*

We can do this alone. But it's harder. So connect. Find someone, or ones who you trust (and make you laugh!)

Sober Podcasts. (Or ANY Podcasts!)

I love podcasts. I love hearing people. I listen to lots–about a whole variety of subjects. A few minutes of tuning in can get you uplifted, give you some motivation, or make your laugh. You can listen to mine of course!

Here's the thing about your sober tool box -you can fill it with all kinds of tools and ideas and plans…..but until you actually USE the tools, ***you're just carrying around a big old heavy box with useless crap in it.***

So What Next?

You have your Sober Tool Box. You've cleaned out all the booze from your house. You are de-cluttering like mad.

And you are getting used to waking up without a hangover!

Before you move onto the next chapter, spend a few minutes answering the following questions and creating your own action plan.

1. Do you know what, when or who your "triggers" are? Identify those cues that prompt your cravings to drink. What are your "rewards"? How can you achieve the same "reward" without the booze?

2. What's in YOUR sober tool box? Make a list of strategies you can use the next time you have cravings.

3. How can you improve your environment? If you haven't done so already, make a plan to get rid of the alcohol in your immediate environment, or ask someone else to do this for you, if it's "triggery".

References

Duhigg, Charles, The Power of Habit, Doubleday Canada, 2012

Chapter 5

Obstacles & Hurdles

The first couple of days of my sobriety was smooth sailing. I wrote this on Day Three.

"Then comes Day Three. It's always the test. I feel like I have purged and cleansed for two days, and to reward myself, I contaminate my body–YET AGAIN–with a bottle of wine,"

It was easy to convince myself that I was *fine,* just being a bit *silly,* after I had managed two days in a row without the booze.

Even with the best planning, the greatest of intentions and a toolbox full of shiny new sober strategies–lots of people don't make it to Day Four.

This chapter is all about stepping into the Arena. Facing challenges, navigating obstacles, and surviving with your sobriety intact.

1 Sober Socializing

If you are going to embrace sobriety, and you prefer not to live in the forest in a hermit's hut, accompanied only by your faithful dog–you had better get used to sober socializing.

The biggest hurdle for many a would-be sober person, is mingling with other people who, at best, will slurp your favourite wine, oblivious to your discomfort, and at worst will try to undermine your resolve.

"What? Not drinking? Don't be silly, one won't hurt!"

Add to that our society's obsession with turning every celebratory event and activity into a reason to drink - ever heard of Beer Yoga? Or Paint 'n' Wine nights?–it's no wonder that us sober "freaks" just want to slink back into our sad, boring cave, and hide under the duvet.

I was faced with my first "hurdle" just seven days into my sobriety. This is what I wrote:

Well we are off for a night camping, and "Before" my only concern would be to make sure we have enough wine. This morning, I have made salad, packed all we need for an evening meal, have fully prepared myself with a cooler full of soft drinks.

We are meeting friends. Camping in Canada usually means lots of alcohol around the campfire. To distract myself, I am taking my fantastic camera (dusted off) to take pictures, as this is a new camping spot for us.

How to Survive Your First Sober Social Unscathed.

 # Plan.

You will notice from the excerpt from my blog (above) that I planned for our camping trip in two ways. First, I had a good supply of non-alcoholic beverages. Second, I packed my camera, so I could wander away from the campfire and take pictures, if it all got overwhelming.

A good plan for your first sober outing includes making sure you have something to drink. You could have a bottle of non-alcoholic wine, or a supply of fake beer, if that's your thing (I often have a glass of fake wine in my hand, if I can't be bothered to explain why I'm not drinking) or at least a beverage you enjoy.

Plan your exit strategy. Driving yourself to the event will do two things–give you a reason not to drink at all and give you the freedom to leave.

Plan to enjoy yourself. I know, this sounds ridiculous..

"I WILL have fun, I will, I will"… because

 # Go with a Smile on your Face

Mindset is everything. If you have already decided that not drinking will mean that the party is as *dull as hell, then not drinking will definitely result in a dull as hell party.*

I used wine as a social lubricant. I thought I was charming and witty when I was inebriated.

Wrong.

I was overbearing, boorish and rude. I repeated myself. I didn't listen to other people. I butted into conversations. I was a drunken pain in the butt.

I also believed I was having fun.

Looking back, I know now I wasn't. I rarely made new friends, and my existing ones drifted away, embarrassed by my behaviour. The only "friends" I had left, were the people who were as wasted as I was. My "drinking buddies".

These days, I love meeting new people. I look forward to social events–not because they are a great excuse to drink–because I meet really interesting people.

I plan on it.

Consequently, I never miss not having a glass of wine in my hand. I'm usually too busy yakking, to notice.

 # Choose Your Events Wisely

When I believed drinking was still "fun", I had an insane fear of missing out.

Any illusion of control over my drinking was swept away, that fateful day when I was introduced to "afternoon wine drinking".

One afternoon, someone invited me over to a friend's house for dinner, with a group of other ladies.

"Come early, around 3 -ish"

And so I did. And was immediately offered a glass of wine.

"Er, now?" I said

" Of course! Drinking wine in the afternoon is lovely…"

And that was that. I had permission. Everybody did it.

By the time dinner actually came, we were all hammered.

The next time I was invited, I didn't get there until about 5 o'clock. And everyone was already wasted.

I felt left out.

So, after that, I always made sure I was around to "enjoy" these afternoons.

But the truth is, I didn't really enjoy them. I knew I would end up drunk. I knew I didn't have the will-power to refuse the booze, however much I intended to. I hated the hangovers; I hated waking up on someone else's couch feeling like crap, and I hated that I would waste the next day getting over my hangover.

But I still did it. In case I missed out. See? Insane.

Now I am not drinking at all, attending one of these afternoon wine fests would be a total waste of my time, and *no fun at all.*

It is possible; I am sure, to only attend social gatherings that are completely dry. But in my world, and I suspect most people's, alcohol is usually present at most events.

I choose to attend those gatherings where alcohol just happens to be served, and I turn down invitations to those socials where alcohol and drinking your face off is *the sole purpose of the event.*

I no longer have FOMO (fear of missing out).

I have occasionally experienced OBIWTGH (out, but I want to go home).

I often revel in JOMO (the joy of missing out).

 # Know it Won't Be as Bad as you Think

Let's put this all into perspective.

I know that it seems big and scary. I know that it worries you that people will stare at you like some sober killjoy. I know that it concerns you that all your resolve and commitment will collapse as soon as someone waves a glass of Merlot under your nose. B*ut please believe me. It won't be as bad as you think.*

I was wound extremely tight as we arrived at the campsite that first sober outing I couldn't avoid.

I was still struggling with cravings, still unsure if this choice I had made would stick, and I was still in daily negotiations with myself on a daily, sometimes hourly basis. So, this weekend was a real test for me in every sense of the word.

Would I be able to get through it without folding? Would I have fun? Would I be the subject of scrutiny, would I have to explain myself.... all of this was at the forefront of my mind.

I needn't have worried. Turned out that everyone there couldn't have cared less what was in my glass. Someone offered me wine, I refused with a simple "no thanks, I'm fine" and the ONLY person who gave any thought to the beverage I was consuming was me!

I noticed another freedom. Because I wasn't drinking, I was not getting irrationally concerned about the amount of booze there was for me and getting resentful if I thought someone else was getting *more* than me.

One thing that people worry about most, is what to *tell people* about the "*not drinking*".

I can tell you I *very rarely get asked.*

Most people, when they are drinking, only care about themselves and their booze. I was exactly like that. I cared about my wine, and it someone wasn't drinking, well, all the more for me!

I only noticed people who weren't drinking when I realized that MY drinking was starting to be a problem. It was then I watched how the "normal" drinkers were behaving.

How bottles of wine went unfinished.

Sometimes even a glass was left half full.

People said… oh no, not for me, I'll stick with water

People said "Thanks, but one's enough,"

The thing is, if your new non drinking status is causing a few people to be curious, chances are that they are feeling a bit concerned about their own habit.

I tell people this:

I quit drinking a while ago. I feel so much better. No, I really need not drink even one. I'm already having fun!

Only occasionally have I come across a negative reaction.

We'll deal with that next.

 # 2 Dealing With the Haters.

"Aha,", said my friend, "I knew you'd start drinking again!"

He was referring to the chilled amber liquid in my glass, which I was enjoying while sitting on my porch step, in the late September sun.

A second later, visibly disappointed when I pointed to the AF beer can, he asked...

"So when are you going to drink again?"

This is a question I am being asked frequently these days. It's as if my friends and acquaintances have indulged this fad of mine for the summer- much the same as indulging a new diet or exercise regime..."Oh God, are you still cutting out bread? One slice will not kill you!" - and are impatient for me to get back to being.... well, the old me.

I wrote this blog post after four months of sobriety. I hadn't declared to the world I wasn't drinking, but it was long enough that most people in my life had noticed that I was not drunk, I had lost some weight, and most significantly, I was refusing wine.

Reactions were mixed. I have categorized them for you, with a short explanation, and some pointers on how to deal with them.

The main point to note, however, is *that most people don't care.*

Category 1. People Who Think It's a Big "Over-Reaction"

Such is the power of the alcoholic stereotype–homeless person living under a bridge, swigging cheap cider, with multiple DUI's and urine stained clothes–that if you don't fit this label, some people cannot comprehend that booze is a problem. A common reaction is

"Oh c'mon, don't you think this is a bit over the top? Why not just cut down?"

The irony is, that if I had announced that I was cutting out gluten, or sugar or red meat, no one would bat an eye.

There are still people in my life who think I am a self–obsessed middle aged woman creating "issues" out of thin air to get attention. These are the same people who think this "fad" will be over soon, and eventually I will go back to drinking.

Arguing is futile. It's a waste of energy.

Category 2. "Normal" Drinkers.

They make one beer last all evening. They have one glass of wine. They are people who actually use those pretty wine stoppers to save the wine after drinking one glass. So they have blank looks on their faces when I try to explain that for me, an open bottle of wine was an invitation for a race to the bottom.

"So why didn't you just stop?" they ask, all confused.

In fairness, the confusion is mutual. I never understood them either.

Category 3. The Actual "Haters"

Rarely will you meet someone who actively works to sabotage your sobriety. But it can happen. One of my husband's business associates still buys me a bottle of wine, despite having been told that I don't drink anymore. A member of my family still refuses to believe I have quit and constantly offers me wine.

This is upsetting, but these "haters" usually have one thing in common–they have a problem with their own drinking. Your lifestyle change has forced them to shine a light on their dark secret. It makes them uncomfortable at best, and resentful at worst. And in order to feel comfortable again, they work to bring you back down to their level.

It's called the "Crab Trap Syndrome".

Bait (chopped up old fish), attracts a crab into a trap. The trap has an opening; the crab wanders in, eats the bait, and then, if the crab is all alone, it will often wander out the trap the same way it came in.

But here's the thing, if there are more than one crab, they will eat the bait, BUT, if one crab attempts to wander out, the other crab (s) will pull it back in!

Even though all the crabs could escape the trap through the opening, they will all prevent each other from leaving. It's the crab version of "misery loves company"

What to Do About the Haters

Avoid these crabs and the bait in the trap.

My advice is the same when you encounter ANY negative reaction to your sobriety.

Minimize contact with these people, establish good boundaries (we will cover this in a later chapter) and carry on in your sober awesomeness.

Some people are just genuinely unsettled by your choices because they are afraid that it will affect their relationship with you.

It is worth noting here that inevitably, some relationships will fall by the wayside. When the fog of booze has lifted, often you find that the 'glue' that kept you together was a mutual love of Merlot.

Digital Detox

Many of our relationships are formed or maintained online.

I personally LOVE the technology that connects me with family and friends on the other side of the world.

But the online universe has a dark side.

You may have wondered about passive aggressive posts about booze and drinking that pop up on your timeline. You may have had people openly challenging you online about your lifestyle choices– often feeling empowered to type comments they would never utter to your face.

You may just get disheartened about the constant "Wine Memes" that circulate through your news feed.

If social media is making you feel anxious, stressed or sad, do the following:

1. Delete and Ban.

Delete "friends" who make negative comments. If they are commenting on a page or in a group you control as an Admin, then delete and ban immediately. If you are not an Admin, then raise the issue with the group leader, and if they refuse to help, then leave the group.

2. Leave Groups.

As much as I loved a Foodie group, the constant references to boozing irritated me. I left that group and found another.

3. Restrict Friends and Family.

I have had to block my sister-in-law from my blog! If banning/deleting family causes more drama than it is worth, then you can manage your privacy settings on most platforms to restrict access.

 # 3 Stereotypes and Stigma

I saw an alcoholic in the bar the other day. She was skinny little thing; she had lines on her face–a typical bar fly; she laughed and joked with the bartender, like a regular. I couldn't see what she was drinking–probably vodka, they always think vodka has no odour, don't they?

It was hard to tell how old she was–maybe fifty? Older than me, I'm sure.

I felt sorry for her. Poor thing. She probably doesn't know any different, probably one of her parents was an alcoholic. They say it could be genetic, don't they? Or maybe there was trauma in her life that can set it off, you just don't know, do you?

You can't help people like that. They have to hit rock bottom, and only then can they turn their life around. But they must go to meetings all the time. For the rest of their life. After all, if you are an alcoholic, it never stops does it? You're always in "recovery". I feel so sorry for people like that, losing their jobs, their marriages. I saw an old tramp sleeping on a bench the other day, I bet he was sleeping off the booze……

Anyway, I finished my wine and went back to work.

I only have a couple of glasses at lunchtime. Wine's not really drinking is it? It's not like the hard stuff. Not like vodka. Gosh, when I go to France, they practically start in the morning!

And anyway, I only drink the good stuff. I never touch that swill that comes out of boxes.

When I get home, I always pour a glass while I'm getting dinner ready.

I love to chop the veg, and sip away, it's so civilised isn't it? And then when the hubby gets home, we have a glass together, and talk about our day. It's lovely to connect over a glass of wine.

I've stopped drinking red wine though. It stains my teeth. I've switched to white. Hubby still prefers red, so I buy a bottle of both, we can afford it, so why not? Sometimes, if I've finished my bottle, I sneak a little glass of red though, it's funny, I always seem to want one more glass…

I'm so tired these days. I so often fall asleep in front of the TV. I can't always remember what we watch anymore! Thank God for Netflix! I can catch up.

Hubby's getting a little annoyed, he has to drag me off the sofa most nights.

We had a bit of an argument the other morning. Apparently, the other night, I posted something silly on Facebook–I must have been messing around with my phone–but I honestly don't remember. He was pretty huffy, I must say, do you know he even said I should slow down on the wine?

Well, I guess he has a point, I got a tiny bit "merry" last weekend when we went out. Not falling down drunk or anything, but apparently I was slurring my words… well I called my friend to apologise, and she laughed and said "Oh don't worry, it's only you being you… the life of the party!"

So I've no idea why he was so mad, you've got to let your hair down sometimes, don't you?

I guess I should try to cut down though. I was late to work the other day; I slept right through the alarm, and then when I got up, all my underwear was still in the washing machine… I didn't even bother to shower, and my head was pounding…

I got called into the Boss's office the other day. Apparently I forgot to file some important papers at the courthouse. Caused a panic… I don't know, I just forgot. Anyway, he was quite unkind, said my work was really slipping.

I didn't get that promotion. Hubby was upset about that too. I don't know; we seemed to be quite comfortable, but my credit card bills have crept up. I was going to pay them off before Hubby found out, but I guess I missed a payment, and he took the phone call…..

Well, that's what's going on in my life. I guess I just feel low these days. I just thought by the time I got to my age, life would be easier, you know?

Well, could be worse, I suppose. I could be like that poor lady in the pub. At least I'm not an alcoholic….

Any of this sound familiar?

There are two dangers of clinging on to this stereotypical notion of the "alcoholic". One is that we don't recognise ourselves, so we go in to a denial about our problem, the second is that we *drink more* to prove that we can't possibly have a problem.

On the flip side of this stereotype is the stigma associated with being sober.

Our society is so saturated in booze, that should you decide to reject alcohol, the assumption is that you *must have a problem.*

So why does this way of thinking persist, even when logic tells us that not all alcoholics are homeless bums and many people choose to live without booze, rather than being forced or court-ordered?

Stereotypes exist when they benefit a particular group of people.

The Alcoholic Stereotype is perpetuated by the Alcohol Industry. They may not have invented it, but they really benefit from it.

For a long time, I listened to the insidious message that the Alcohol Industry whispered to me…

"You don't want to be the other… a "raving alkie", a weak, pathetic person who can't hold your booze. You don't want to be part of that club…. keep drinking… you're not like those people"

And so I did. Until one morning, I looked in the mirror.

I saw a middle-aged bloated woman, flushed with dark circles under very sad eyes.

And all I wanted, was to wake up in the morning, and know what to say to my husband. Because, yet again, I had gone to bed drunk the night before, and although I was fairly sure we had made love, I had no actual recollection.

So I joined the "others", in that sober club that terrified me. And found out all the members were just like me.

I finally began to heal.

One of the hardest aspect of quitting booze is feeling like you no longer belong. That you are one of the "others". And any negative reaction to your choice may reinforce that feeling.

I wish I could tell you that there is an easy solution.

But there isn't. You have to join the club. Become one of the "others".

And only then will you realize that you are one of the lucky ones.

Chapter 6

What to Expect

As soon as you quit drinking, you can expect no hangovers and zero drunkenness. OK, that's obvious, here are a list of changes I experienced in the first month.

Better Pooping.

Why is this top of the list? Not just because I'm British and we're famed for our toilet humour… no, this improvement will make you feel significantly better. Not to cast too much of a light on this subject, but if you have been straining out stone hard marbles (due to being chronically dehydrated), interspersed with the… erm… exact opposite, a healthy bowel movement is cause for much joy. Not only does this mean that the horrible bloated feeling will recede, it also means that your body is slowly adjusting to being… well, normal again.

Better Sleep.

News Alert! Alcohol does not help you sleep. Passing out does not count as sleep at all. Alcohol will initially make you drowsy, but a few hours later (when you're supposed to be in your deepest, most important sleep cycles), alcohol will wake you up, torture you with shame and humiliation, and refuse to let you get any rest. Thus, in the morning, not only are you dehydrated and hung-over, you are also suffering from sleep deprivation.

It takes a few nights before you get back into a healthy sleep rhythm. For the first alcohol free nights, you might experience some insomnia, but bear with it, soon you'll be back to sleep, glorious sleep.

The Kitchen Is Clean (er)

The next worse thing after waking up with a hangover, is to face a kitchen with last night's dirty dishes all over it. Drinking in the evening ensures that stuff does not get done. I'm not Suzy Homemaker, but these days, fifteen minutes of cleaning up after we've eaten, makes for a joyful morning…….as does….

Never Running Out of Clean Underwear.

Small domestic chores often get disregarded when we're drinking, because, well, that would cut into our Wine Time, wouldn't it? Many is the time I overslept (or lay in bed, hoping that my headache would recede), skipped the shower, only to discover that my underwear was either in the laundry basket or going moldy in the washing machine where it had been for three days…. yes, I admit, there were times when I had to sort through my cleanest dirty underwear, to avoid being late again.

(Almost) Never Being Late….

Because I now have a more organised laundry system, plus I sleep better, plus I don't have to face a filthy kitchen in the morning… means that far more often, I am on time for appointments. This also means I am not so much of a liar. Which is also good.

Remembering TV Shows.

I relied heavily on Netflix to not only show me what we had been watching but also providing me the opportunity to watch it all again. Thus (while I was in denial about my "problem") allowing me not to make slip ups, like making my husband sit through several movies twice, because I had no recollection at all, of ever watching them before.

Less Insane Social Media Updates.

Drunk Tweeting. Drunk Facebooking. Drunk texts. Drunk emails. Thank God I never got my head round Periscope and Facebook Live wasn't a "thing" while I was drinking.

More $$$

If you drink one bottle of wine a day, depending on your tastes, you could be anything from $100 to $300 wealthier in just ten days. Minus what you spend on cake. But it's still good, my friends, and it only gets better!

Better Teeth.

This is important to me, because as an English person living in North America, I get a lot of flak about my teeth. Which are fine, I might add, but I am not obsessed with having "Osmond family" pearly chompers. However, due to a nightly bed routine, which is not just falling into bed and passing out, I do pay far more attention to flossing, cleaning and yes… whitening…

Better Skin.

I left this to last, but for me it one of the most noticeable and welcome improvements, I've always hated my skin, and while I was drinking, I hated it more. I was flushed, often sweaty, and had developed patches of rough flaky skin around my nose and forehead.

We all acknowledge the damage that alcohol does to our liver, but the skin is an important organ too, and I abused mine, by forcing it to work overtime, trying to flush poison out of my body.

I still don't have beautiful skin, but it delighted me that the flushed look had gone, and I looked clearer, in only ten days after I quit booze.

Pink Clouds.

What is a Pink Cloud?

The term pink cloud, according to AA, tends to be used negatively to describe people who are "too high" on life, after becoming sober. They are described as people who have lost touch with reality and are now living in a fantasy land. The emotions that these people experience do not properly align with their actual *life*.

Well, that sucks.

Basically, if you are feeling great for the first time in decades after quitting the booze, someone saying you are on a "Pink Cloud" is metaphorically wagging their finger and whispering…. pride comes before a fall.

The implication is that this happiness is a sign of over-confidence, and the recovering boozer is just heading for a weekend binge, induced by euphoria.

That's a little dramatic.

Enjoy the Joy.

It wasn't until I quit drinking I realized how miserable I had become. Drinking had first masked some problems I had (real and imagined), but eventually had compounded them.

When you quit drinking, all your problems and issues and difficulties are *still there. They didn't magically disappear.*

For the first month or so of quitting drinking, I revelled in my newfound sense of well-being. It felt a little like I was convalescing after a long illness (which, in a way, I *was*). Every day I would get a little stronger, get through cravings a little quicker, and face a new situation without the booze.

I did this by focusing on the positive improvements of sobriety.

It was a little easier to resist a craving if I could conjure up the pleasure of morning coffee with a hangover.

MY pink cloud moments were more like silver bullets of positiveness, helping me punch through moments of frustration and doubt.

There are ups and downs. And sometimes…… nothing.

"I woke up this morning feeling....... nothing. How weird. Over the last 10 days, I have been waking up feeling elated that I didn't drink the previous day... And regardless of how I have felt physically, emotionally and mentally I have been cheering and doing handstands (in my head). But this morning...flatness. Of course, I have only really experienced depression, shame, grumpiness, and self- loathing in the morning, along with queasiness, sweatiness, and bloatedness (not sure if that's a word), for the last fifteen years, followed by the aforementioned elated and happy feelings over the last ten or so days, so this nothingness was a surprise,"

I am sad? No. Happy? No. Angry? No...... Just flat.

Is this how "normal" people feel?

One thing that drinking had successfully obliterated for me was the ability to sit through unpleasant feelings.

Feeling sad? Pour a glass of wine.

Lonely? Let's have another.

Angry or hurt? Wine, now.

But booze had also killed off the joy. I lived for pleasure only.

I filled my pink cloud with small moments of *actual happiness.*

I still savour the moment when I wake up in the morning, without an impending sense of doom, just joyful anticipation of the day ahead.

With every Pink Cloud, however, a little rain must fall.

Hippos and PAWS.

One of the numerous reasons that finally compelled me to quit drinking for good, was that I was scared shitless about the number of blackouts I was having.

Not the woozy memories that come back in embarrassing flashes of you dancing on the table, or doing embarrassing Karaoke, no, I mean the total loss of memory.

I still have no recollection of seeing some movies, I have no recollection of making phone calls, posting on Facebook, sending emails - only the horror of the evidence the next day, or the confused and irritated texts from friends.

At the end of my drinking days, I would have complete blackouts of conversations and situations, even after drinking just a few glasses of wine. It was not uncommon for me to have no memory of getting to bed. I would wake up at 3.00am, dehydrated, depressed and frantic that I was losing my mind.

Recently, scientists have found the reason for these blackouts. It's both a vindication for me, and frightening to think of the permanent damage I may have done, had I carried on drinking.

It's all to do with your Hippo.

That's correct. The Hippocampus. Australia's National Institute of Alcohol Abuse and Alcoholism (NIH) released their research on the connection between alcohol and blackouts. First, they found that women experience blackouts more frequently than men, and with less alcohol.

Your Hippocampus (Hippo) lives in your brain and is a recording device that stores all your memory data. When you hose down your hippo with booze (as I did daily), you stop the recording process. But already recorded memories, up to that point, remain.

Therefore, I can remember the start of many evenings, the first couple of glasses of wine then..... *nothing.*

The Hippo can recover - for a while. At some point (and scientists don't know when) damage becomes permanent and also starts to affect the rest of the brain. Scientists also don't know the reason it gradually takes less and less alcohol to black out more frequently.

But should that matter? If we blackout once, even twice, isn't that a wake- up call? Shouldn't we listen to our Unhappy Hippo?

Stupidly, I took far too long to care for my floundering Hippo. Luckily for me, there seems to be no permanent damage - except to the unhappy recipients of my alcohol induced communications, and my own embarrassment.

But every so often since I quit drinking, I have had a few days when my brain seems really foggy; I feel tired and lethargic–sometimes even flu-like, *almost like a hangover.*

When it first happened, it was a surprise. Until then, being sober meant that my energy levels had increased, my sleep was refreshing–I could say I was dancing on my Pink Cloud! And then, suddenly I wasn't bouncing like Tigger, I was moping like Eeyore.

Not only that, I was really forgetful.

My fear was that my poor hippo had suffered permanent damage

Thankfully, I discovered, that all these symptoms were normal and had a cute, cuddly name–PAWS (Post Acute Withdrawal Syndrome).

These symptoms, which can be really debilitating ,are the body and brain's way of re-setting and re-wiring if you like. It's as if the brain powers down to do a regular maintenance check and some tweaking and adjusting.

The bad news is that these symptoms can continue up to two years after you quit, at regular intervals.

As time passes, the good news is that the symptoms get less intense.

A bout of PAWS, if you're not prepared, can lead to a relapse. In fact, it's been recognised as a leading trigger for picking up the bottle.

For me, being informed was the biggest defence. Recognising the symptoms, knowing they will pass– making sure that all my self- care routines are in place, being as gentle with myself as my daily routine will allow–ALL these things got me through my bouts of PAWS.

I look at it like this. I welcome PAWS. It means that I'm healing. It's like when you have a cut or a wound and it scabs over and heals. You get an annoying itch, and the temptation is to scratch and pick at the scab. But you know this will mean that you potentially can open the wound again and your healing will go back to square one.

This is how I view PAWS. That itch means that my unhappy hippo is adjusting to life without booze, my body and brain are healing and improving. My only job is to let nature take its course.

Nostalgia.

"Nostalgia - it's delicate, but potent. Teddy told me that in Greek, "nostalgia" literally means "the pain from an old wound." It's a twinge in your heart far more powerful than memory alone. This device isn't a spaceship, it's a time machine. It goes backwards, and forwards... it takes us to a place where we ache to go again. It's not called the wheel, it's called the carousel. It lets us travel the way a child travels - around and around, and back home again, to a place where we know we are loved"

Don Draper, Mad Men.

Visualize yourself with friends on a sunny summer afternoon. Three of you enjoy a chilled glass of bubbly.... you've got so much to chat about, your families, your careers, and you re-live all those memories from when you were are college together... you order another bottle... let's celebrate our friendship!

It's Christmas Day. All your family is around you! The kids have opened their presents, Hubby is carving the turkey and you all raise a glass of wine...Merry Christmas!

Ahhh, it's so beautiful, the sun sets over the vineyard and you bask in the warm Californian evening... a second honeymoon. You chink glasses and drink to your love...... So Romantic!

Nostalgia is a beautiful thing, like a benevolent "Ghost of Christmas Past". How about a touch of "Harsh Reality?"

After your third glass of bubbly your lips are loosened somewhat, and you reveal to one friend, that her best friend slept with her boyfriend at college. Unfortunately, her best friend happens to be the third friend sitting at the table... an argument ensues, you gulp down another glass, and break the heel of your shoe as you hurriedly depart.......

Christmas Day. You are hung-over from the night before; the kids were fighting because they had to wait for you to get up before they could open presents; the turkey is overdone, and you're hammered and passed out before the Queen's speech. Hubby has to clear up the kitchen and is pissed off.... Merry Christmas...

You drink a glass or three too many at the Winery, so any continuation of your romantic evening is out of the question.... or was it? You can't even remember getting to bed......

Nostalgia. Big fat Liar.

Feeling nostalgia for our drinking days can be a dangerous trigger.

I try to recall my drinking days in the same way I think of past relationships. After all, there were good times and laughter.

I remember a warm summer evening with friends, all of us drinking. I remember Dexy's Midnight Runners playing in the background, and I can still hear the laughter as we all sang tunelessly to "Come on Eileen".

I can smile at that memory and still know I have moved on, and can never recreate that moment.

Even amid my darkest drinking days there were moments of fun and laughter. Nostalgia allows me to remember those.

In the same way I can feel a fondness for an old lover–even though the relationship was toxic–but never want to rekindle the flames, I can look back at the fun part of my drinking days, and never want to relive them.

The Addictive Personality.

Ice cream.

Cake.

Sugary Sodas.

Shopping.

Shoes.

Junk food.

Filling that wine shaped hole was all I could think about when I quit. I *needed* ice cream. I *craved* fake beer. I was unsettled and distracted myself by downloading novel after novel onto my kindle. I binge watched Netflix.

The concern is that we will simply replace the old addiction with a new one. It worries us that we have a personality disorder or a disease which will just manifest itself in a gambling casino or with piles of pizza boxes.

This is normal.

There is no scientific evidence for the *'addictive personality'*

What we are looking for is another distraction from our life. Something else to give us instant gratification. We are looking for that moment of pleasure, of numbness from our problems–a way to forget.

I had forgotten, if I had ever really known, that happiness differs greatly from pleasure. Happiness takes time, of course, and some effort. I had gotten used to the "instant fix".

Now I didn't have the booze in my life, I would have to work those sober muscles, and find my happiness.

Chapter 7

Sober Muscles

There's a big difference between getting sober and living sober. The former requires focus, effort and venturing outside your bubble into the "uncomfort" zone. It also requires self-awareness. The latter is when your "uncomfort zone" is your new normal.

In the previous chapter, we talked a little about the difference between "normal" drinkers and "dysfunctional" drinkers.

For me, it was all about HOW and WHY I drank that differentiated my boozing from "normies". I didn't like myself very much. I felt itchy and scratchy in my own skin. I wasn't happy with my career, my relationships, my achievements (or lack thereof)–I wasn't happy with any of it. But instead of tackling this head-on, I played the victim and drank to escape.

Getting sober was only the start for me. Staying sober and doing the work necessary to finally feel comfortable in my skin meant that I had to create a life that supported my sobriety and my happiness.

I dislike the concept of "living in recovery". It sounds *stuck*. For the same reason, I don't identify myself as an alcoholic.

My goal was (and is) to live a full and vibrant life in sobriety. As a non-drinker.

To achieve that goal, I use my four "sober muscles".

Whatever stage you are at in your sober journey, you need the energy to keep going. To keep walking down that sober path. So it pays to be in good sober shape, to have those sober muscles all toned up and able to carry you through the up and downs, over the rocky patches.

That's why I spend time every day, working out those sober muscles.

 # Sober Muscle 1 Self- Care.

The first Sober Muscle is Self-Care.

When I was drinking every day, I truly believed I was "treating myself". Wine was my reward, was what I was working towards each day.

That first glass of wine punctuated the end of my working day and the beginning of adult relaxation time. Wine, I believed, *was my self-care.*

When I quit drinking, this self–indulgence filled me with guilt. I was horrified about the time wasted; the money spent and friendships squandered. So the last thing I thought I deserved was more *self-care.*

I couldn't have been more wrong.

Over the years, I had been in destruction mode, and now it was time to get back on track.

A common misconception about self-care, is that it's all about pampering yourself. I would get visions of "wellness retreats" and spa days, or hours spent getting my hair and nails done.

True self-care is far removed from this.

It requires self-awareness and some real work. Self-care leads to self-love. One of the greatest achievements of anyone's life, is the ability to look in the mirror and love the person who is smiling back at you.

So how do we get there?

I focused on four areas–physical, mental/spiritual, social and purpose.

Physical Self Care.

It sounds self-explanatory. Who doesn't know that we are supposed to eat "properly" and exercise regularly, right?

Problem is that most of us focus on weight management rather than physical wellness. We despair of our curves and bulges, our dress size and the number on the scale, and abandon any notion of nourishment.

It's not our fault.

We've been conditioned to despise "fat".

Love Your Body.

In my late twenties, I dated an older man, and then stayed with him for fifteen years.
He was obsessed with my weight.
"You're the fattest girl I've ever been with"… he said once, almost in bewilderment. It was true. I had seen pictures of his ex's, and I knew his ex-wife. They were all very thin.
I wasn't huge, but I was certainly a "solid build".
That comment stayed with me, and because I was young and stupid, and he seemed experienced and sophisticated, my mission in life was to transform my "solid" body, into a sleek, streamlined machine. With muscle definition.
I started running obsessively. This was OK because Older Man also ran obsessively too. So I entered my miles into a training log, I watched calories (fuel, not food), I measured my waist, thighs and monitored my heartbeat and pulse rate.

And I hated every minute.

I even 'competed' in lots of races. Marathons (London, four times), half marathons and 10k's.
And throughout the entirety of our relationship, Older Man referred to me as "chubby". Not as a description. *As a name.*
Interestingly, when I look back at those fifteen years, although I wasn't drinking to excess (too many calories), I was having to "control" my drinking.

For instance, I would never open a bottle of wine before eight or nine at night (so I would go straight to bed afterwards instead of opening a second bottle–it wasn't a fool-proof method). I would measure the glasses of wine out *exactly, so I got my exact and equal share, and sometimes I would sneak a gulp out of Older Man's glass if I got the opportunity.*
When the relationship was over, I stopped running and started drinking.

And here's the bizarre part……… *I got thin!! I dropped about 20 pounds!!*
I existed on Wine and Toast.

The reason I was thin, of course, is that I was stressed and malnourished.

Gone was "chubby girl" and in her place was "Booze-chic girl".

I went from one extreme to the other and I still hated my body.

It wasn't until I quit drinking I began to accept and celebrate my body. It took baby steps.

Addition, not Deprivation.

I threw away ALL my diet books. Every. Single. One.

I eat ALL food groups–yes, even carbohydrates. I eat a varied diet. I eat cake and pizza and salad and quinoa. I don't "demonize" food. It's not "good" or "bad", it's just food.

If I listen, my body will tell me what it wants. If I stuff myself with pizza and junk for days on end, my body signals by becoming bloated and lethargic–that it could do with a salad, thank you very much.

If I'm hungry, I eat. When I'm full, I stop. If I'm bored, sad or emotional, I stay away from the fridge.

We all have unique bodies with different nutritional needs.

Over time, my body weight has stabilized. I only know this by the clothes I wear, I don't own scales anymore. I'm not the same weight at fifty-ish, as I was when I was twenty, and I'm OK with that.

Get Moving

So this is how I used to exercise; pound my body for an hour or so, in the gym or the pool (swimming used to soothe my hangovers) and then lounge on the couch the rest of the day, glugging wine, convincing myself that I "deserved" the booze.

This is not the way to exercise sensibly.

Our bodies were made to move. Consistently.

I walk most days for about an hour. It's inexpensive and easy to fit in. And I also keep active. I garden, I take the stairs instead of the elevator; I have been known to ride my bike, and I regularly join up with friends for a hike, or to go fishing or anything that doesn't just involve sitting on my backside.

Get a Sleep Routine.

Lots of us don't get enough sleep–hint: passing out from too much booze isn't sleeping.

Alcohol will make you drowsy at first, and then will wake you up. Hence the passing out on the couch, followed by stumbling to bed, fitful sleep and then waking up at 3.00am, unable to stop your mind whirring. Followed by a day plagued with the hangover AND sleep deprivation.

I existed like this for over a decade.

Imagine my joy when I first woke up, *after a full eight hours*, feeling refreshed, energetic and hangover-free.

It takes about a week before your body adjusts to being free of the alcoholic "sedative" it was used to. But hang in there, and you will rewarded.

To help along your healthy sleeping habits, I suggest;

1. Don't drink coffee or tea just before going to bed (unless it's caffeine-free)

2. Don't eat just before going to bed.

3. Go to bed and get up at the same time everyday

4. Don't have a TV or electronic devices in the bedroom.

5. Keep your bedroom well ventilated.

Mental and Spiritual Self Care.

There are many people who experience a spiritual 'awakening' when they quit drinking. Once they are free from their addiction, they find themselves drawn to a less materialistic and "consumption–based" existence. Some people work through the Twelve Steps and reconnect with God.

But none of this is a mandatory part of getting sober.

Mental and spiritual self-care for me is three things: living in accordance with my values (integrity), learning to value myself, and living in the present.

These all help me be comfortable in my skin.

Integrity.

Now "integrity" is a word that's banded round a lot. We think of business people has either having integrity or not for example. We also bundle together "integrity" with trustworthiness and honesty. All good traits obviously. But living a life of integrity for me means living in harmony with my values because if I don't, I feel discord and unease. It's interesting that I saw a saying recently, "When your heart and your head disagree, your liver always suffers"….. and this for me is true.

So sometimes it IS easier to take a shortcut, and rationalize to yourself that something is OK, when in your heart you know it isn't–well that makes me unhappy. So "walking the walk" may mean more inconvenience, but it brings peace and lasting happiness for me in the end.

Validating Self-talk

We all tell ourselves stories. We tell ourselves stories about our failings, our flaws, about what other people think about us, about what terrible things might happen in our future because of our failings. We get so mired down in our stories, that we believe them, they become part of our identity, and they become self–filling prophecies. Because the stories and fantasies we built in our mind influence our reality. Our stories directly affect our behaviour. I'll give you an example. I had a boyfriend once, who was very insecure. He didn't believe he was worthy of being loved. He thought for sure, once the first romantic flush of a relationship had worn off, any woman he was with would see him for the worthless person he was, and leave him. None of this was true. He was a sweet kind man. But this insecurity affected his behaviour. He so believed I would eventually leave that he behaved in such a way as if I were leaving. He became angry and suspicious; he questioned my every move; he was miserable to be around. Eventually I left. There was no way the relationship would work, unless my boyfriend could work through this story he had told himself, and see it was just a fantasy. His story instead became a self-fulfilling prophecy, and the consequence was that the end result validated his story.

So we have to be careful of validating our stories to ourselves. If we are constantly telling ourselves that we are failures, we are not enough; we aren't smart enough, not responsible, whatever our story may be….it affects the way we behave, and becomes a viscous circle.

Part of my daily self-care, is to question my stories. Ask myself, is that true? What evidence do I have for that? Is this story helpful? Or is this story harmful? How can I re-frame this?

Living in the Present.

We can become too obsessed with the past. Especially if there are moments of cringe-inducing humiliation embedded in your memories that leap out at you when you least expect it. And I should know. I've spent many a dawn hour, re-living and re-hashing.

Learning from your past is great. Living in your past is not.

To help me put all this stuff to rest, I wrote about it. Some is forever private, and some you can read about in Sober Ever After. Once it was all down on paper, I got rid of the stuff I didn't want "out there" and the rest I published. And made peace with the Ghost of Jackie Past.

Now, my past is a learning tool. Nothing more, and nothing less.

I believe no one can really avoid periods of self-examination as we journey down the sober path. And that's healthy. But just remember, if you are constantly checking the rear-view mirror, you will miss the beautiful scenery.

Sweating The Small Stuff

Self-care isn't always the fun stuff.

I am a procrastinator. If I allow myself, I will put off doing small, inconvenient tasks for as long as possible.

Errands such as sorting our bill payments, reconciling the bank account, returning forms, making phone calls to difficult clients–all the annoying administrative tasks that most of us need to do, so that our lives run smoothly.

If I am not careful, these small tasks will pile up.

And then I get completely overwhelmed and stressed.

I used to drink to ease my stress. It never worked, because once I stopped drinking, my stress and all those undone tasks were still there.

Part of my self-care routine for my mental wellbeing, is to do these small tasks *as soon as I possibly can.*

I sweat the small stuff.

Social Self Care.

Ahh, we don't do all this sober self-care stuff in a vacuum. There are always other people to contend with.

To look after myself, and protect my (healthy) relationships, I had to do two things–stay away from drama, and erect boundaries.

Stepping Out of the Drama and Creating Boundaries.

Let's be clear what we mean when we say Drama

"Drama" I define as a situation or incident that could be very easily resolved by two or more people communicating calmly and reaching a consensus, or at least an understanding of each other's point of view… but instead, is escalated into a negative, angry conflict, devoid of any reasonable communication, usually with one or more parties determined to play the role of the victim.

Drama is energy draining, negative, time consuming, tiresome…. and if taken to the extreme, damaging to your relationships and sometimes, your health.

So why do we (because, I'm betting that YOU, like me, are NOT innocent here), why do we take part? Or even instigate drama?

Well, for me, most of my drama originated when I was drinking and involved me in a starring role as the victim of some perceived wrongdoing, or something I felt should have been done or said, but wasn't… ALL completely in my own mind. And in hindsight, my impulse to play the victim, came from me not liking myself and hating what I was doing to myself. Creating a drama with me as the persecuted one, in some twisted way rationalized my behaviour. *It gave me a reason to drink.*

If people are so mean I have to drink right?

People tired of my drama. They were fed up of my self-pitying posts on Facebook, my drunk texts and my self- righteous emails. Most reasonable people drifted away from me.

So, when I quit drinking the first behavioural modification was to address the drama. And the first way to do that was to start communicating clearly. And this meant working on my boundaries.

I was always a people pleaser. I wanted people to like me, therefore I would say and do stuff that I thought would "make" them like me. Trouble was that this didn't always work, and I ended up doing and saying a lot of things I didn't want to say or do. And then I would get resentful. And then I would assume the role of 'victim'.

This had to change.

When someone asked me for something, instead of saying YES, when I wanted to say NO, and then bitching away, (probably to someone else) about the thoughtlessness of this poor person who should have the temerity to request something of me, clearly not CARING how busy I was… thus making myself both a victim AND a Martyr in my Drama Scene….. I said NO. No drama, no victim, proper adult communication.

The first step to eliminating drama in my life, was to eliminate my own.

The second step is to eliminate everyone else's…. the drama you are sucked into, that intrudes into your life, and takes precious time away from you leading the best, most inspirational creative sober life you possibly can.

This is a little harder.

Communication is one key as we have mentioned.

Identify the Drama Creators around you. They are EASY to spot. They are the people who are always the *victim*–always in a negative space, - always, or nearly always complaining about their lot in life–and (often) wanting to gossip in a mean negative way about other people.

Hold people like this at "arm's length", if you cannot eliminate them entirely from your life.

Check your social media and restrict people who love drama. You don't have to block them, just don't get their notifications.

Other Energy Drainers–as I call them–are the people who request your ear, or your shoulder to cry on. They want your help and advice yet refuse to do the work to help themselves. This kind of drama is subtle, but drains you, nonetheless.

These are not the people who genuinely seek your help and advice, or just want a little moral support. The Energy Drainers will constantly complain about their life, often blame other people and will ask for your input, again and again.

But they will never DO anything to change. They will never take heed advice. They will never try to change their circumstances. They will never be accountable for their actions.

These people are stuck.

If you let them, these people will suck you into their negative vortex, and will keep YOU stuck if you're not careful.

And if you are doing all the hard work that sobriety entails, you need every ounce of positive energy you can get to keep moving forward.

Looking After Your Purpose.

This is the last of my self-care objectives, but arguably the most important.

What could be more sacred than finding your purpose in life? And then working to align with it and achieve all your dreams and goals?

For many years I felt like a fish out of water. I was in a "career" that I didn't love, I felt trapped by debt and helpless to change my situation.

Feeling powerless changed to feeling resentful. And rather take responsibility for my life, I expected other people to 'save' me. And when they didn't, I blamed them. And I drank. A lot.

The drinking numbed my disappointment.

I can't pinpoint the moment when it changed. It was a whole series of events and situations that lead first to putting down the bottle.

As the fog cleared, it became plain that "if it is to be, it is up to me". I alone am responsible for my choices and decisions.

Being accountable to myself has been the hallmark of my sobriety. No more blaming, no more playing the victim. No more waiting for someone else to ride in and save the day. No more manipulating.

Gradually I have been able to change my direction in life. I wanted to write, so I sat down and picked up a pen. I wanted to be creative, so I experimented and tried new things. I wanted to be in charge of my financial destiny, so I immersed myself in our business and made a plan to pay off debt.

It didn't happen all at once. Sometimes even the baby steps are more like a shuffle forward. *But at least it's always forward.*

Sober Muscle # 2–Creativity.

I haven't got a single creative bone in my body.

At least, that's what I used to tell myself. And believe.

"I'm not creative, I'm a numbers person. A science person. I don't waste my time with fanciful notions of creativity–I put away those childish things–literature, poetry, dance, art, inventions……..you name it, I'm not good at it, and if I'm not good at it, what's the point of doing it?"

What a sad state of affairs. Yet, I'm betting that I'm not the only one who is carrying around these limiting beliefs about capacity to create–and I bet those beliefs have no basis in reality.

It's so often that we think we can only focus on activities in our life that lead ultimately to *achievement.* We put such great emphasis on "success". And we abandon all those things we just do because we like doing them.

Drinking is the opposite of creativity.

Drinking dulls the mind, atrophies the brain, diminishes our energy, and sucks away our motivation. Think about the "activities" that you used to do while drinking. If you were anything like me, you had a MILLION fabulously creative ideas half way down a bottle of Merlot, which evaporated into thin air before you reached the bottom on the bottle.

It's not for nothing we have the saying–Genius is 10% inspiration and 90% perspiration–that's what creativity is. We can only focus and perspire and stick with these amazing ideas if we are sober.

So here's the other aspect of creativity–it's not just the expansion of our abilities and pushing the boundaries of what we perceive are our limits–it's the PROCESS of creating that really protects our sobriety.

Psychologists have discovered that it's not the result that causes the greatest happiness, but the process. So I really encourage you all to make bad art. Every day.

Sober Muscle # 3–Gratitude

Want to be happy?

Count your blessings. Be thankful.

Misery comes from focusing on what we perceive to be lacking in our lives.

Grateful people live in abundance.

Grateful people are not victims.

In his book, 'The Happiness Advantage" the psychologist Shawn Achor says:

"gratitude has proven to be a significant cause of positive outcomes. When researchers pick random volunteers and train them to be more grateful over a period of a few weeks, they become happier and more optimistic, feel more socially connected, enjoy better quality sleep, and even experience fewer headaches than control groups"

Living in gratitude not only supports my sobriety and helps prevent a relapse; it allows me to embrace my sobriety as a blessing.

Sober muscle # 4 - Connection.

In the early days of sobriety, my social circle shrunk. By my own design. Some people I hung out with– well they are perfectly lovely people, but our main connection was a shared worship of Merlot, and I no longer worshipped at that altar.

I also found that my true self wasn't really as extrovert as I had been acting out for the last years.

My introvert self didn't mind hanging at home.

But no person is an island, and even the most introverted of us needs human connection.

Johann Hari argues that addiction results from disconnection.

While I personally believe addiction is multi-faceted, loneliness seems to be a factor.

At the time when my drinking was at its heaviest, I was alone. Having moved to another country, and then split up from my long-term boyfriend, it disconnected me from my entire support network.

Wine became my companion.

I sat alone in my apartment most evenings, sipping on a glass of wine, until a bottle (or sometimes two) was empty.

Drinking alone compounded my loneliness. I wasn't motivated to try to meet new people; I got used to sitting on the couch with my chardonnay.

The only people I associated with, were those who also drank like me. I didn't have friends; I had *drinking buddies*.

I found my new tribe on the internet.

When I started blogging, I connected with the online sober community. Over the last couple of years, I have made some of these connections in person.

I have also strengthened ties with my family–even over long distances!

Shame over my drinking meant that I really turned inward.

Breaking the vicious circles of loneliness–drinking-more loneliness isn't easy.

It starts with putting down the booze and then continues by nurturing the relationships you have and stepping out of your comfort zone to create new ones.

The most powerful connection I have made has been with myself. A self- awareness I didn't have before. Time to acknowledge thoughts and feelings I have and then work through them, rather than smother them, or avoid them, or transfer them onto other people.

I've found a new self- respect. I'm respectful of my emotions. Anger, sadness, joy…. all those emotions happen for a reason, and they are all equally important. So they all deserve the same respect. No emotion or feeling is wrong.

Working out my sober muscles is a daily habit. The main purpose is to support my sobriety, but my sober muscles also help me *be happy*.

For a long time, I wasn't sure what happiness was. Like many people, I had confused "pleasure" with "happiness".

Pleasure v Happiness….

Everyone who has slumped down into the couch after a long day, and taken a swig of chilled chardonnay, or has scoffed a large bowl of Hargaen Daz ice cream can tell you what pleasure is.

Tt's that moment of euphoria, where you slip momentarily away from your troubles, into a warm and fuzzy state.

Those moments are usually short-lived. And so we chase them, again and again.

Who remembers that the second glass of wine was never as satisfying as the first?

And that–right there, is the very definition of addiction–constantly grasping after something that is always just out of your reach.

One of the worst habits we have to break, apart from obviously the actual drinking, is this need for instant gratification.

We live in a world now that worships instant gratification. We have instant entertainment, instant information, fast food, instant connection…….. and therefore our values and our sense of wellbeing have got well, *skewed.*

We are mistaking PLEASURE for HAPPINESS.

We want shortcuts to feel good. And that is (I believe) just as hard an addiction to break, as the actual physical, chemical dependency we have on alcohol.

This isn't new. Human beings have been looking for the quick fix of instant pleasure and the problem as I see it, is that we confuse this with our quest for happiness.

Our overall goal as human beings is to seek happiness…. this isn't just a tag line for beauty pageant contestants, it's a recognized purpose of human life, from as far back as Aristotle. If we needed any further endorsement, we can look to the American Declaration of Independence that lists the pursuit of happiness right up there with liberty and life itself.

But, anything worth having, is worth working for.

First, we get this happiness thing all the wrong way round. We think if we have the RIGHT job; we are the RIGHT weight; we get the RIGHT partner– then and only then will we be happy.

OR, we think happiness should be somehow "provided" to us by the other people in our lives.

Happiness is something we create ourselves. And that takes work and some time rather than the quick fixes we have been used to.

Psychologists have done experiments with kids–offering them ONE chocolate bar right now, or if they are prepared to wait…. THREE chocolate bars in a few hours.

Children overwhelmingly choose the ONE chocolate bar NOW.

This is very much like the "drinkers" response to pleasure. We want it now. We want the instant "fix" of that glass of wine.

Dependency on this pleasure fix is an immature as a child wanting the chocolate bar *right now.*

In many ways, when we put down the wine, we finally start to grow up.

In the same way that children want us to wipe their tears, we as drinkers shy away from any feeling of unhappiness.

We hate those uncomfortable, inconvenient sad moments. We loathe feeling low, and all scratchy in our own skin. We want to fix that RIGHT NOW.

When I first lived on my own, I hated it. I loathed being by myself. Being responsible, not only for all the practical things in my life but also being completely responsible for my own emotions. There was no one else around me to blame for my sadness or my loneliness–and no one to complain to either! So I made friends with wine. And together we sulked away evenings.

But I wasn't any happier. And I wasn't any likely to GET any happier any time soon… and I imagine that for the few number of brave souls who took the time to care about me, I wasn't a lot of fun to be with.

It wasn't until I took responsibility for creating my own happiness that things got better. And it didn't just instantly get better just by putting down the bottle either. Please don't get the idea that happiness will miraculously "appear" once you take away the booze. There's more work to do.

Exercising those 'sober muscles' is a great start. It helped me transform myself from that kid who wanted a chocolate bar RIGHT NOW, to a (more) patient, mature person who knows fleeting pleasure will be gone as quickly as I can chomp down a chocolate bar, whereas the happiness I create and nurture lasts forever.

Embracing Sobriety–Working Out Those Sober Muscles.

Incorporating self-care, gratitude, creativity and connection into your life takes time and practice. I suggest picking out one or two daily exercises at a time and seeing what works for you. And then you can tweak and adjust!

Here are some hints to get you started.

- ☐ Pick one physical act of self-care daily. It could be going for a walk, drinking a few glasses of water, getting an early night.

- ☐ Do a "digital detox" and unfollow the "drama queens" on your social media.

- ☐ Count three blessings every day–they could be as simple as the smell of your fresh brewed coffee in the morning.

- ☐ Call a friend and get together for coffee.

- ☐ Instead of turning on the TV, work on a creative project. It could be cooking a new recipe, reading a new author, or starting a DIY project you have been putting off.

References
Achor, Shawn "The Happiness Advantage" Crown Business, 2010

Chapter 8

Relapse

I cannot write a 'how to' book about quitting drinking without mentioning the dreaded "relapse".

You may have heard the phrase, "relapse is part of recovery"

I call Bullshit.

Relapsing is *not inevitable*. It does NOT have to be part of your journey.

Now, before you write me furious emails, let's take a step back and examine exactly what a relapse *is*.

What is a Relapse?

I define a relapse as slipping back into old patterns of drinking for a prolonged period.

So a relapse is NOT (in my view):

Slipping up and having a glass of wine with dinner.

Having a few drinks at a party.

Drinking occasionally on holiday.

I don't believe you are in "relapse mode" if you slip up. You hit a few road-bumps.

This does not mean that you should be complacent about slip-ups!

On the contrary, if you have given in to a craving, or pressure from other people then it's time to revisit your sober toolbox (see chapter 3).

What you shouldn't be doing is beating yourself up. Or starting at "Day One". Or blowing this all out of perspective.

Treat this as a warning flag.

And remember this:

"Slip ups are part of recovery," (see what I did there?)

So, What is a Relapse?

A relapse happens when you ignore the warning signs of your slip up. A relapse is:

Persuading yourself that having a glass of wine with dinner is fine

Getting drunk, or deciding that it's OK to "let your hair down"

Telling yourself that holidays don't count.

Augusten Burroughs defined a relapse like this;

"A relapse is the temper tantrum you allow yourself to have when you forbid yourself from drinking..."

The difference between a slip-up and a relapse is *mindset.* A slip-up can happen in a split second moment, sometimes without you even realizing it.

I have been handed a glass of wine (without being asked if I wanted it) and have just stopped myself from taking a swig, not because I wanted it, it was like an involuntary reflex. I didn't drink the wine, but it was a reminder to be on my guard.

Relapsing can result from the following:

Missing Ground Work.

"I wish I could wake up in the morning and not want to drink,"

So say all of us. But that is not how this works. In order to not want to drink, you have to not drink, and enjoy not drinking. Rinse and Repeat.

Skipping the first inconvenient and uncomfortable bits will not get you to the "not wanting to drink" part.

The inconvenience of removing alcohol from your environment, the uncomfortable moment when you inform appropriate people you're not drinking, changing your routine and scheduling time for self-care.

It's all essential. And if you miss this part, you'll make relapsing a probability rather than just a possibility.

So many relapses occur because people try to quit in secret, and then their nearest and dearest–none the wiser–purchase the usual box of wine for the weekend.

"This time," someone emailed me recently, "I'll be honest with my husband I've quit for good"

Self-Fulfilling Prophecy.

If you EXPECT to relapse, you WILL relapse. If you listen to that little negative voice that tells you you ALWAYS fail at this kind of thing, you have NEVER been able to accomplish anything, so why BOTHER about this sober thing…. is it any wonder that this kind of negative self-talk results in a drinking splurge?

Resentment

"It's not fair!"

Like a toddler having a tantrum, we focus on the "treat" that is now denied to us.

We live in a state of deprivation, and inevitably, a prolonged period of jaw-clenching *every time someone else gets to have a drink* becomes too much to bear.

"I'm an adult! I'll drink what I want!"

Sabotage

"Go on, just have one,"

Our need to fit in, coupled with the confusion of our friends and family, often leads to relapse.

This new sober role we have taken on, feels strange and uncomfortable to *everyone.*

Unconsciously, we try to make ourselves and others "feel better", so we sacrifice our sobriety.

The Rebound

For a slip-up, there is only one course of action–get back on the wagon immediately. You run the risk of a slip-up becoming a full-blown relapse if you delay.

"I'll start again on Monday", is "relapse thinking" and should be a red flag (unless today is Monday).

The Blame Game

Of course, don't beat yourself up, it's a total waste of energy.

But blame no one or anything else either.

How do I quit the booze if my husband/boyfriend/significant other insists on drinking wine? How can I do this if he/she isn't supportive?–is a regular lament I receive.

One lady wrote to me;

"My husband still uncorks a bottle of red and pours himself a glass to have with dinner. He doesn't seem to get it–the rest of the bottle just SINGS to me for the rest of the evening… but he won't stop. It's causing arguments, what do I do?"

OK, disclaimer here–I'm not a marriage guidance counselor. In fact, I have two failed marriages behind me, so I'm probably the last person in the sober universe you should ask for relationship tips.

However, I do have a (very supportive) husband who still drinks occasionally, and (so far so good) we still get along, so here's three things to consider before you make an appointment with the divorce lawyer…

Are you giving out "mixed signals?"

I tried to moderate for about three years before I finally quit for good. It's well documented–my good intentions and epic failures. Every week, I would give myself a stern talking to and make a big announcement to my bewildered husband, that THIS TIME, I was really serious. And I forbade him from bringing home wine. Or cider. Or anything that I could be tempted with. On lots of these occasions, I would also couple this with a new diet, and a new exercise regime.

Inevitably, after a few days, I would be a wine - deprived, carb–starved raving psycho!

IF YOU LOVED ME YOU WOULD GET ME WINE!!

The poor guy didn't know what to do. Did he remind his hysterical wife about all the BIG PLAN to not drink alcohol until Friday night? Or did he dodge the flying bread knife and run down to the store to get Wine and chips on Wednesday night and restore calm to the household?

Most of the time, he got wine for me.

It was a lose-lose situation.

You could argue that he was "enabling me". But honestly, the poor man just wanted peace and quiet.

When I did finally quit, I didn't even tell my husband for about a week. He clearly noticed, because not only did I not purchase wine myself, I also refused a glass… on a Friday night!

If any of this sounds familiar, the lack of support you are feeling from your husband or partner, may result from you crying "wolf" too many times.

So focus on doing the sober work YOURSELF….
and you may see that gradually your partner realizes that this isn't a fad–it's serious. And then you can discuss ways they could help. Or join you!

Working on Your Mindset.

"Today will be a great day, if you choose not to be a miserable cow," Facebook Meme.

I took a long time to understand that my "mindset" is not something that happens *to* me, it's not the result of some mysterious outside force, it is a *daily choice.*

I can choose to be happy. I can choose to be grateful. I can be a victim of life, or I can make lemonade with those darn lemons.

I know, it sounds a bit "Pollyanna–ish".

But it's true.

Avoiding relapse, and making your sobriety "stick" successfully, at the intersection between self-awareness and mindset.

At that pivotal point, remember this mantra

"If it is to be, it is up to me"

Steps to Take Immediately After a Relapse

Immediately. *Immediately.*

1. Self-Analysis.

If you are British, like me, then "self-analysis" is a hyphenated swear word.

There is nothing I loathe more than uncomfortable navel gazing. So I feel your pain. But suck it up buttercup, because if nothing changes, then everything stays the same, and if you have read this far through my ramblings, then I know you want your life to change.

Ask yourself the hard questions.

Are you doing the work?

I've said it many times–you can't manifest sobriety. It takes work. It takes planning and strategy.

Do you have a fridge stocked with alternative non-alcoholic beverages you can drink while your partner sips on wine?

Have you got a book to read, a project to work on, a sober blog to write if you are hearing the Wine Witch whisper in your ear?

Are you making the choice to take a walk? Or meditate?

Or are you setting yourself up to fail?

2. Adjust Your Plan.

So it turns out that visiting with your BFF on a Friday night is a huge trigger because she refuses to believe you have quit.

So, *don't go.*

Counting sober days, instead of motivating you, has become a crushing, overwhelming pressure.

So, *stop counting days*

Your favourite Fake Beer, is your favourite because it reminds you of the real thing. AND has you craving for the real thing.

So, *drink sparkling water.*

You can change the tools in that sober toolbox. You can tweak your plan.

3. Change Your Mindset.

As I said above, Mindset is a choice.

Try to look at sobriety as a gift you give yourself on a daily basis. It is hard at first, you DO feel you are depriving yourself–but make a physical list of all the reasons you quit booze in the first place–and then another list, where you jot down ALL the benefits of sobriety. The thing is that second list keeps on growing. Keep it with you, in a notebook or on your phone and refer to it regularly. Keep on adding to it.

4. Focus On Today.

Relapse is often a response to overwhelm.

"OMG, this is forever,"

No, it's not. It's for today. Everything we have is just for today. So just don't drink today.

Asking For Help.

The biggest blessing that my blog The Wine Bitch bestowed on me, was a tribe of sober cheerleaders. Complete strangers reaching out through the Sober Cyberverse to commiserate if I felt low, to cheer if I was having a great day, or if I had an "aha" moment, just noting their agreement, or putting forward a point of view I may not have considered.

Johann Hari wrote in his book "Chasing the Scream" all about the necessity of having a tribe.

"The opposite of addiction is not sobriety. The opposite of addiction is human connection,"

While I believe addiction is far more complex than this appealing soundbite, I can confirm from my own experience, that having a tribe of friends (even virtual friends) who "get" what you are going through, helps you along this sober journey.

I mostly attribute my lack of relapses to the hours I spent online, reading blogs, leaving comments and sharing my thoughts with the sober world.

As time has passed, my tribe has expanded.

Far from being socially isolated because I'm a *boring sober person,* I have many new interesting people in my life, who do not give one solitary shit about the beverage in my glass.

How did I find this tribe?

I paid attention.

From my self- analysis (shudder), and observations, I understand now, how inward–looking and self-absorbed I had become. At social functions, I was more concerned with the availability of booze and how much I could consume without being noticed. I gravitated to the "drinking crowd" to mask my habits.

I didn't spend much time listening to anyone. I avoided the people who weren't drinking, *in case they judged me* and consequently, my social circle was made up of drinking buddies, who validated and encouraged my boozing.

My new tribe isn't new at all.

They were there all the time. I just never paid attention.

Non Alcoholic Activities.

Alcohol is everywhere. On the TV, in the pub, in other people's homes–I wish that everyone in the world would realize how awesome life is without booze. But I also wish I could have a pink furry unicorn kitten for a pet. And neither is likely.

These days, I see flyers and advertisements for "Beer n Yoga" and "Paint n Wine Nite".

It does feel like every activity has been hijacked by Booze.

Even toddler's birthday parties seem like an excuse to uncork.

So it does require effort to find activities that are not solely focused on getting wasted.

It sounds clichéd, but filling your time with something you love doing, WILL help prevent a relapse.

You have to fill that Wine Shaped Hole in your life, with something you enjoy *more than Wine.*

For me, it was gardening and writing. For you, it might mean photography or painting. Or studying to change careers. Or training for your first Ironman. Or sewing your first quilt.

The trick is not to force it.

The trick is to allow your passion to find you.

References

Hari, Johann "Chasing The Scream" Bloomsbury Publishing, 2015

Summary of Part Two

- Getting started requires taking action.
- The Big Secret to sobriety is to stop drinking – everything else is a strategy to help, not a "magical cure"
- Planning is a key strategy
- Plan to remove alcohol from your environment, adopt an "alcohol policy" and tell someone your plan.
- Have a strategy for cravings – Distraction, Escape, Acceptance
- Focus on breaking the habit.
- Identify your "triggers" and "cues' and change your "routines".
- Establish a Sober Toolbox, comprising substitutes for booze, projects and calming activities.
- USE your Toolbox!
- Hurdles to be faced include Socializing, "Haters' , "Stereotypes and Stigma"
- Planning and strategizing using your new tools can overcome all these hurdles.
- There are (good) physical side effects from quitting booze.
- A Pink Cloud is the euphoric side effect from quitting.
- PAWS is the less pleasant effect.

- Nostalgia can trip you up if you are not careful
- Sober "Muscles" can help you – if you work them out daily
- Self-Care, physical, mental, social, and purpose is one sober muscles
- Creativity, Gratitude, and Connection are the other three
- Finding a way to work the sober muscles on a daily basis will help you start to LIVE in sobriety.
- There is a difference between "slip-ups" and a "relapse"
- A relapse is sliding back into old patterns and mindset
- If you do relapse, examine the reasons. You may have to revisit some of the groundwork
- If you relapse, or slip up, it's important to start again immediately.

Part Three

Sobriety, Tools & Transformation.

"What you get by achieving your goals is not as important as what you become by achieving your goals"

Zig Ziglar

Chapter 9

First, Make Your Bed.

In the first weeks of being sober, it was as if a veil had fallen from my eyes. I looked around my house as if I were seeing it for the first time. I noticed all the undone or unfinished tasks–stuff jammed into drawers and closets, disorganized piles of paperwork, clothes in heaps. Not to mention the spare bedroom that had become a receptacle for all the junk I couldn't be bothered to deal with. Some parts of my house looked like an episode from "Hoarders"

Don't get me wrong, we weren't living in *absolute* squalor; I had just been doing the bare minimum to keep the house clean and habitable.

The clutter and disorganization made me anxious. But now I was sober, I couldn't deal with the anxiety by having a large glass of wine. So I dealt with the cause.

Over a few weeks, I de-cluttered like a madwoman. I got rid of recycling, old clothes (donated), I shredded old paperwork, cleaned out closets, and dealt with my fridge that resembled a scientific experiment.

It was extremely therapeutic. Not only did I have a huge sense of accomplishment, it also focused me on a task (which hadn't happened in a while) and it kept my mind off the "Wine Witching hour".

I then turned my attention to my much neglected business. Here too, I had been getting by doing the bare minimum. So I decided to undertake the "Great Business De-clutter"

I cleaned off my desk. I went through every piece of paper, and I either "junked" it, filed it away, or put it on a "to-do" pile. I overhauled my complete filing system, and re-arranged my filing cabinets, so I could actually find stuff when I needed it. I even changed the office furniture around so I wasn't in danger of a broken ankle by tripping over cables and wires. I put up an inspirational poster and cleaned off my white board.

My physical Inbox and my electronic Inbox both were ruthlessly purged. I went through my emails and deleted all the old ones. I electronically filed the others. I "Unsubscribed" from any email list that didn't add value to my life–most of them! I answered the most pressing ones.

I did the same to my physical Inbox. I only left tasks that were urgent and relevant to my business. If they were "nice to do" tasks, I filed them away, if they had been in my in-tray for over six months, I threw them out.

It left me with a small pile of correspondence and tasks that needed my attention

Last, I de-cluttered my software.

In desperation, I had tried all kinds of software and applications that promised to "magically" solve all my business problems–everything from bookkeeping to making me coffee in the morning–and I used hardly any of them! So I cancelled all but the platforms essential to the running of my business.

Let me be clear, none of this magically solved all my Big Hairy Assed Problems, like my Debt, or my much depleted client list, but the first step radically improved my confidence and my sense of control.

After decades of drinking, my pile of "small stuff" had snowballed into "big stuff".

"I'll get back on track tomorrow" was my mantra, but I drowned my good intentions every evening with wine, and somehow the days all seemed to fade away without me ever finding the "track" to get back on.

The wine could never quite numb the guilt, or occasionally the panic, as I failed to call back clients, finish work on time, or file my tax returns.

It was a pattern of Procrastination–Drink–Guilt–Drink–Failure–Drink–Stress-Drink, with an overall sense that storm clouds were gathering, and sooner or later, my world would implode.

So I drank some more.

My first manic weeks of de-cluttering were more than just a distraction. It felt like I had pressed a "Reset" button.

Sweat The Small Stuff.

Focus on the BIG PICTURE! Challenge yourself! Don't Sweat the Small Stuff!

I felt overwhelmed. How could I pay off debt and make my business a viable, successful venture if I couldn't deal with a kitchen sink full of dirty dishes or make my bed?

The solution? *Make my bed.*

And after that, clean the kitchen.

Sweating the small stuff–*literally just focusing on small achievable tasks* - was not only the start of cleaning up the wreckage left from my drinking, but also the start of my sober life.

Somehow, making my bed on a daily basis was helping me maintain my sobriety.

The Disaster List

The little problems don't go away. They fester and rot and eventually infect your life.

After pressing that reset button, I knew I couldn't slide back into old habits; I had to capitalize on this small, unfamiliar sense of self-worth.

I made a Disaster List. Sounds dramatic? I could have called it a "To Do" List, but somehow that didn't capture the urgency I felt to get my life back on track. My *sober* life.

The list included the big stuff that caused me most stress. Unfiled tax returns, paying off debt, unfinished client work, *getting more clients,* and then the smaller, but no less important tasks like getting the car serviced, basic maintenance on the house… all the way down to clearing off the recycling from the back deck.

It was a long list.

Eating An Elephant.

How do you eat an elephant?

One bite at a time.

I took tiny, tiny steps.

I divided the bigger stuff into smaller tasks.

For example, one day I printed off all the forms I needed to fill in for my tax returns, and just completed the easy stuff that didn't need thinking about. The next I gathered up all my receipts. The next day I made an appointment to file…… it took a few days, but the crossing tasks of my list each day kept me going. Gave me some confidence.

It felt like I was moving forward a little.

I tried to get into a routine.

Mornings were hellish when I was drinking.

"You lie in bed this morning, waiting for the nausea to pass and imagining your demise. You hear your husband grind the beans, the clicking of the gas stove as he heats water. And then, fifteen minutes later, you smell the coffee. Your cue to get up,"

Apart from the hangover, and assessing how much damage control would be needed for the rest of the day, my mornings were noteworthy for the complete lack of routine and order.

I left the house, late, sometimes wearing yesterday's underwear, mostly without eating properly, and always with a throbbing headache.

It was never a good start, and so many times the morning shambles set the tone for the rest of day.

Routine, although much maligned for being *boring,* was my saviour. *Routine, far from being stifling, set me free.*

I didn't have to worry about clothes, files, a to-do list for the day, because part of my routine was (and is) to take a few minutes at the end of each day to make a checklist of essential tasks for the next day, and any appointments, get papers and files ready so I wasn't rushing around, and rummaging through drawers and desk, and to make sure I had clothes ready.

I also cleaned the kitchen each night, so I didn't face an overwhelming mess in the morning. I went to bed *at the same time every night, in the bed I made first thing in the morning,* and I set the alarm.

The result?

A calm, relaxing morning, time to drink coffee, catch up on the news, knowing that I was fully prepared for the day.

The impact of the rest of the day?

I didn't feel "on my back foot" and defensive

I could navigate my way through daily 'disaster' without becoming enraged.

I wasn't wishing that the day would end *so I could drink.*

Some Bites Don't Taste Good…

Procrastination is often born out of fear. And on my "Disaster List" were many items I avoided doing because I was fearful or ashamed, mostly around the financial situation I was in.

Making a phone call to creditors, or *even people who owed me money*….. filled me with dread.

These were the bites of the elephant that were not appetizing at all.

Remember when your mum wouldn't let you eat dessert until you finished your greens?

I could only gag them down by holding my nose and *just doing it.*

This is the way to deal with the stuff that scares you.

1. Do it first.

2. Hold your nose.

3. Endure the taste–it's never as bad as you think

4. You'll feel so much better afterwards and can reward yourself with the "easy" stuff.

Every day I made myself do *at least one horrible task.*

And remember this–most nasty tasks start out quite palatable, they only start to fester when they are *ignored.*

One Big Hairy Assed Problem–Debt

I've never been great with money.

I don't gamble or anything, and I try to pay bills on time and *not* rack up debt, but it always appears I should do better than I really am, I should have a savings account, I should not have a credit card debt, I should have a plan for my retirement…. but none of these things are so.

Money just seems to vanish.

I try to get better.

I try to make a plan, write a budget, keep tidy files, and save a little money every month. It works for a while, and then I slip back to doing none of those things.

I purchase on impulse. Stuff I don't really need.

I have habits, like buying a takeout coffee instead of just brewing my own, downloading a new book to my kindle, shopping for ingredients for one meal, instead of looking in the fridge and creating a meal from the perfectly good food I already have. I occasionally forget to transfer money to our joint account, so a payment bounces and it costs $48 extra, because I wasn't organised enough.

I put my head in the sand and think…" I'm not that bad"

Any of this sound familiar?

My relationship with money has been much the same as my relationship with booze.

I work on a "moderation" budget…. and then I get visited by the "Fuck It Fairy" and I blow my plan. Again and again.

I hope that someday I will magically win the lottery, but I know, in my heart, that if I did, I would be one of those people you read about after a big win–who blow it all, and end up living under a bridge.

The worst thing/best thing about quitting drinking for me, was that all my "money issues" came sharply back into focus.

No longer was I able to avoid and deny and numb the stress I caused myself by NOT dealing with my finances.

So I started the struggle down the path of financial sobriety. There have been some detours, but the general trend has been forward.

Debt is one of the main causes of stress. If your drinking has been triggered by stress, then here are some of my tips to help navigate through this Big Hairy- Assed Problem.

#. Know Your Numbers.

Remember when you were in denial about how much you were drinking? This is the exact same issue. Denial will not help you out of the financial hole. Take a deep breath, and write down ALL the debt you have–overdue bills, car loans, personal loans, credit cards, money owed to friends and family, child support, unpaid taxes, unpaid mortgages. EVERYTHING.

Then add it up.

It's just a number. Numbers can only hurt you *by surprise.*

Once you know your Debt Number, calculate your Income Number. Again, everything including your salary, income from your business (after business expenses), rent income, rent from offspring, tax rebates.... everything.

Then calculate your living expenses. Rent, Mortgage, utilities, car expenses, food, clothing, etc.

 # Know the Solution is Simple (but not easy)

Just as weight loss is as simple as calories out versus calories in, debt piles up when we live beyond our means, or we have unexpected expenses that result in more money going out than coming in.

Debt repayment starts when we can reduce our outgoings or increase our income.

Go back to your daily expenses. Where do you "leak" cash? What money do you spend that you don't *need* to?

Here are some examples:

Takeout Coffee

Takeout food.

Magazines (printed or online)

Clothes you don't need.

Garage Sales

Gym Membership you don't use.

Online Subscriptions you don't use.

Bank Charges for bounced cheques, or monthly charges that could be re-negotiated

Insurance policies that could be re-negotiated

Cable bills for channels you don't watch

Food you purchase but don't really need.

Booze

The last one is really important. Put aside ALL the cash you used to spend on booze and allocate it towards paying off debt.

 # Can You Increase Your Income?

Can you work some overtime? Can you take on a second job? Is there someone in your household who could contribute a little more? Do you have unwanted stuff you could sell?

Allocate any increase in cash to paying off debt.

 # Talk to your Creditors

I know you don't want to. But I promise you it's easier to make the phone calls, than to *avoid the phone calls.*

Ask for realistic payment plans.

If you need help, find out if you have organizations in your area that can help you.

NOTE: Look for government-approved agencies that SHOULD NOT charge you for their services. BEWARE the scammers.

 # Prioritize Your Debt Payments.

First, you should focus on the debt that is most urgent. So mortgages or debt re-payments that will keep a roof over your head, or your car on the road so you can get to work, are the most important.

After that, experts will tell you to pay off the debts with the highest interest rate first.

I didn't do that–I paid off the smallest debt first. It gave me some confidence, and a feeling of progress.

Keep Track.

I have a folder (a new one each month) for all my monthly bills. I list all my obligations on the inside the folder and cross them off as they get paid. That way, I never miss a bill, and I avoid any unnecessary bank charges for returned payments.

Keep Going

Once you have paid off your first debt–don't go out and blow the cash! Roll the extra money over and pay off the next debt quicker.

Have Strategies.

Know the difference between "want" and "need", and question yourself when you feel the urge to shop, or that impulse to purchase.

"Do I really need that?"

"How will I feel if I buy that?"

So many of my shopping expeditions–so called "retail therapy"–have been blighted by my buyer's remorse afterwards. The quick "fix" of pleasure dissipates soon afterwards, just leaving me in a state of guilt and further in debt.

I tackled this in a familiar way, devising strategies and tools for my Financial Sobriety.

1. Knowing My Triggers.

In the same way I had to identify the times and situations that prompted my drinking, I developed self-awareness around my spending. The result? Unsurprisingly, I over-spent when I was feeling lonely, stressed, or bored.

2. Distraction.

When I found myself in one of my spending states, I distracted myself with free activities–a walk, gardening, a few minutes of meditation–until the "craving" to go shopping, passed.

3. Focusing On the Positive

Being grateful for what I had, finding joy in simple things, and pride in small accomplishments meant that I learned to live without "stuff". I adjusted my values.

The Corrosion of Consumption.

Remember a few chapters back when we were talking about Pleasure v Happiness? How, as drinkers, we were looking for that instant gratification, the immediate 'feel good" moment?

Over- consumption is the same mindset.

New car? Exotic holiday? Or something smaller– new furniture, or expensive trendy food to impress your friends? Our impulse to purchase is often driven by the need to get a quick "gratification" fix, not unlike that "need" for a glass of wine.

When you first living in financial sobriety, it's not uncommon to get push back from people close to you.

We live in a society infected by the Booze and Consumption paradox.

We are encouraged, motivated, *shamed* into spending more and drinking more. Our generosity is measured by the amount of money we spend, in the same way that our sociability is judged by the beverage in our hand.

Yet, when it all goes wrong, we are often rejected.

Debt and Alcoholism are viewed in the same way– *personal failures. Being broke or in debt is an embarrassment. Not being able to "hold your booze" is the same humiliation.*

The biggest lesson of getting sober–both from booze and financially–is that neither consumption of material "things" or booze is necessary for happiness.

There is a serenity and freedom that comes when you realize that you don't have to buy a new car if the old one works perfectly well.

There is a sense of pride that comes from recycling, or saving up for something, instead of paying by credit card.

Once you can reject the notion of "more", or measuring your self-worth by the value of your possessions, life becomes a lot less complicated.

I'm not saying it's easy–the path to financial freedom can be as rocky as the sober one–but the journey is worth it.

And remember this:

Money doesn't make you happy. But paying your bills does.

Chapter 10

Sobriety Becomes a Tool

Sobriety is not a destination. It is not even a journey, *in the end.* Although it is a way of life or course, it is also a tool for life.

Everything I have learned, all those knocks and bruises and stumbles–all of that I use and apply every day.

From getting out of debt (see last chapter) to running our business, there is not a single situation that doesn't benefit from the lessons of sobriety.

When I was quitting, I had a business. It was a reincarnation of a couple of previous ventures that had failed.

It was a tough path and still is.

Conventional wisdom says *don't make any big decisions during the first year of sobriety.*

It's a vulnerable time. Would it have been easier to find a nine-to-five job and just concentrate on my sobriety? Probably. But that's not a luxury I have, unless I want to uproot and move to Alberta, or a bigger city where there are decent higher paying jobs (but not many affordable places to live) and then there's the unavoidable truth I am just about fifty years old, my qualifications are outdated and I'm set in my ways unemployable)

And, more importantly than that, I know that life is short (I learned the hard way, after drinking away the best part of a decade), and I refuse, just refuse to spend another minute, in a soul-destroying office, waiting for the weekend.

So I choose entrepreneurship. And I believe now, after struggling through the difficulties of sobriety, whilst hanging on to the rollercoaster ride of operating my own business, that my sober journey has made me a better business owner and has significantly contributed to the progress I have made.

Whether you own your own business, or you are trying to make your mark in your own career, don't think about your sobriety as an obstacle–embrace it as a tool to help you.

Here's how:

People already think we are weird.

Remember all those times when people said "Oh, come on, you can just have one drink right?

And remember all those people who, instead of being supportive, took your sober lifestyle choice as a personal insult?

Welcome to entrepreneurship. Welcome to the career ladder.

In my life, there have been two times when I really felt I was the "black sheep"–when I quit drinking, and when I started my own business.

On both occasions I was at best misunderstood, and at worse, ridiculed.

Conversely, on both occasions I discovered the true generous hearted cheerleaders in my life.

In sobriety, you have already experienced the sense of not belonging.

So now, don't be defeated by those who try to sideline you. Revel in being a maverick, an "outlier". It's a good thing. You're changing the world!

We understand the concept of Progress, not Perfection.

The path to sobriety is littered with obstacles. We remember well the "slip ups", the relapses that came out of nowhere. We know not to beat ourselves up, just pick ourselves up and keep going.

When things go wrong, we've learned to regroup, to try another strategy, another angle, until we achieve our goal.

We are not held hostage by the concept of perfection. We know that is an ideal not a reality.

We recognise and celebrate progress and keep our eyes and focus on the horizon ahead.

We've turned our destructive behaviour into Creative pursuits.

Firstly, it was a necessity. We needed a distraction. We needed projects, for those times when the Wine Witch came calling.

But after a while, we discovered "creative flow". We mastered new talents and skills.

Since I've been blogging, I've met ("virtually") sober crafters, writers, carvers, musicians, life coaches, artists, and horticulturists.

We've dispensed with the Myth of the Drunken Tortured Creative Genius.

Since quitting booze, I've not only had a myriad of ideas, (that I remember), I've also been able to think myself "creatively" through business issues, and occasionally turn problems into opportunities.

We know the value of money

Because we've wasted so much of it. It's been estimated that even a "normal" drinker can spend up to $100,000 in a lifetime.

Since I've been sober, I've invested $9000 (so far) that I would have spent on wine, either into my business ventures, or paying off debt.

So we know the power of spending only what we have, and the perils of over-consumption, just to make ourselves feel better.

We know the Value of Time

Again, because we've wasted so much of our precious time on either swilling booze on the couch watching TV, or recovering on the couch in front of the TV.

I estimated when I quit that I had wasted approximately 23 months of my life (over the last decade of drinking).

Every moment is precious. We know that now. We use our time productively, and constructively.

We understand that communication and integrity are the basis of good relationships.

We've had to face unpleasant truths and communicate them. We've had to apologize. We've had to convey our feelings. We've had to stand up for ourselves occasionally.

Cultivating good relationships, whether they are with customers, clients, staff or co-workers is a skill is as essential to building a good business or career, as it is to maintaining our sobriety.

We know the importance of healthy boundaries.

I took a long time to say "No" and not feel bad about it.

Now, I say it regularly. I also turn off my phone, shut down my email and social media whenever I start to feel overwhelmed.

I've also learned to not waste vital energy bandwidth on people who don't deserve it, people who drain my energy without giving back. I've blocked, deleted and restricted people without a twinge of guilt.

I focus my energy and love on the positive people in my life. Whether they are friends, family or clients.

We know that it's not weak to ask for help and support

At the beginning of sobriety we know nothing. It's common, though, for our ego, in an attempt to hide our fear, to show up as arrogance, and pretend that we know everything.

Soon, however, the flaws in this plan show up. We have to look for support (and find it) in online groups, via sober bloggers, AA meetings, SMART meetings, podcasts… anywhere that other people who have experienced, or are travelling the sober path, hang out and generously share.

As there is no place for Ego in sobriety, there is no place for it in entrepreneurship. In both situations, we are continuously learning.

We know how to look after ourselves.

Self care is vital. We have to eat healthy food, maintain sleep and exercise routines, meditate, make time for fun and love.

We must make time to replenish our soul, our creativity, our mental health. We cannot give from an empty cup, in sobriety, in business or in life.

Using the tools we have gained during this sober journey, is almost the pinnacle of this Sober Pyramid.

But there are a couple of things we haven't yet talked about.

Higher Power.

If you read lots of sober blogs and articles, they may persuade you that you are not "doing sobriety right" if you are not drinking green tea, attending yoga regularly….and don't forget about that spiritual epiphany!

It's unnecessary to suddenly take on a new religion or spiritual practices just because you have quit drinking.

When I first quit, I was willing to give anything a go. Green tea, green smoothies, rubbing crystals, chanting at the moon, 'releasing ceremonies', playing Pan's Pipes… literally anything.

What I was trying to do was find some peace from the constant chatter from the Mind Monkey in my head. And if aligning my feminine energy with the North Star would shut that fucker up–even for a few minutes–it was worth a go.

So I went from a fairly healthily skeptical person, to embracing full on witch-hood. It was a confusing stage of my sobriety for everyone, including me.

So did it work?

Well, yes, and no. So here's my take on everything woo woo and the benefit to my sobriety–and then you can make up your own mind.

1. Manifesting and the Law of attraction.

In the most simple of forms this means that "you attract what you put out". So if you project happiness and light out to the universe, you'll get more of the same back, and if you are a miserable cow, then you'll get plenty back to keep you miserable.

There's definitely (in my experience) much benefit from the power of positive thinking. Happy people are more likely to be successful and rewarded by opportunity. This isn't just "woo woo", science backs this up also–read The Happiness Advantage by Shawn Achor.

However, just transmitting happy thoughts out to the universe won't make you sober. "Manifesting sobriety" just doesn't work–I've tried. You just don't wake up one morning with all your urge to drink just "manifested away" by the Universe. You have to stop drinking and experience all the cravings and nastiness that comes with it. But, if you focus on the positive benefits of sobriety more often than whining and moaning about how deprived you are, it's more likely that the sobriety will stick.

One last note about the Law of Attraction. Some people get freaked out about every negative thought–as if the Universe will punish them with everlasting torment. It doesn't work like that. You're allowed to feel grumpy and blue, that's normal on this sober journey. If you plaster on a cheery smile, and are continuously perky, it will make people like me, (who doesn't really give a flying f*ck what the universe thinks) want to punch you.

2. Meditating.

There are lots of bullshit woo-woo stuff around meditating. It's all about calming your soul and quietening your mind. You do not have to drink green tea beforehand (or any time, for that matter), you don't have to sit cross-legged on a mat; you don't have to chant. You can do guided meditations if you want, or pray, or listen to "spa music", or you can go for a walk, or have a bath, or garden, or clean the toilet. It's about clearing your mind. There are no rules.

3. Crystals, Tarot Cards and Astrology.

I love all the above. They are a great distraction. The crystals look pretty. But again, they do not ward off the demon drink. Tarot cards may help you think a little differently than usual–but they will not "predict" how your sobriety will end up–only you can do that. Please don't email me about chakras and crystals. YOU STILL NEED TO DO THE WORK (see above re Manifesting).

Spirituality and connecting with your Higher Power can come from simple things like gardening.

I used to hate gardening. Until the day when I particularly nasty craving came over me, early in my sober journey.

In desperation I went out into the garden, (ignoring the bugs) and started tearing out weeds…… I just physically jammed my hands into the dirt to stop them picking up my car keys and going out to buy wine.

It worked.

So I did it again. And again.

By then I had cleared quite a patch, and then my husband gently explained that they weren't all weeds…. so we spent an hour re-planting.

And then I was hooked.

Since then I have acquired a greenhouse. Someone was throwing it away, and my husband rescued it and re-built it for me. He built me EIGHT raised beds. And then a Gazebo. Last year was my best harvest so far (although I couldn't figure out the problem with my tomatoes and I grew about fifty pumpkins… who knew they would all "take"?) and this year I am being far more adventurous.

Now, instead of a bottle of wine, my husband brings me new plants… A Miniature Kiwi! Raspberry Bushes! A Lemon Tree! I am giddy with delight.

Every morning, I check to see how my seedlings are doing, with my coffee in my hand. In the evenings, with dirt under my nails, I have my tea, or an NA beer under my Gazebo.

Life has changed. I have changed. I'm more concerned about the planet and our environment (never crossed my mind while I was drinking), I think about stuff when I am planting. I feel more connected and yet "freer" if that makes any sense at all….

I found my Higher Power in the garden.

Helping Others.

One of the core philosophies of AA is that of "Addicts helping Addicts".

At first, coming out of the "sober closet' is daunting, not just because of possible negative reaction from others, but also the potential impact on those around us.

I am lucky. I am self-employed and all my wonderful step children are grown up, so I was not afraid to be "Sober Out Loud". There were no repercussions from co-workers, or other parents.

Not everyone is in an ideal situation.

But you can still help others.

Be a Lighthouse.

Shine the way for others.

It is unnecessary to tell your story or give explanations. It's not even required to give advice.

You can set a shining example without making any grand announcements about your sobriety.

For Friends…

Since I quit, I have found that many of my social circle have also quit or substantially cut down. At first it concerned me that they were only doing this out of politeness, but when I asked one friend, she said

"I noticed how happy and healthy you looked. So I thought I would give it a try"

For Family…

Our children learn from us.

My step-grandchildren were exposed to "Drunk Grandma Jackie" far too often.

Many sober bloggers have reported that not only are they setting a far better example for their children, they are also "present' in their lives.

It's not "cool" to be a Merlot Mum. It's damaging.

For Strangers…

Writing a blog or a book, even with a pen-name can help others. Telling your story whenever you can is a powerful tool. You never know when you will touch someone else's life, say the one thing that changes everything for them.

The power of words can save lives.

Chapter 11

Full Circle

Hey you!

Yes, you with the glass of wine in your hand!

No, I haven't got magical powers, and this book is not equipped with a teeny spying gizmo, I just know myself, and I wasn't that different from you.

I flirted with sobriety for a long time before I committed to a permanent relationship. And while I was flirting–I carried on drinking.

I read many books about drinking and sobriety with a glass of wine in my hand.

At first I read them because I was looking for signs I was different. *Special.*

But I'm not special and neither are you.

Research is Fine.

I love research. It makes me feel I am productive, even when I am not producing a thing. It was a great delaying tactic.

I read lots and lots about getting sober. I mostly read it in secret, hiding the covers of books or my tablet, not wanting anyone to question why I was reading do much about quitting booze.

If I research the crap out of this, I can delay actually doing it.

There's Nothing New Under The Sun.

If you have been reading this, hoping for a "miracle cure" or a "quick fix", then I am sure you are disappointed.

There are no short cuts and there is no way to get sober *without actually quitting drinking.*

There is no way around this simple, straightforward fact.

If you want to be sober, stop drinking.

Stop Thinking and Reading and *Do.*

Get out of your head.

For the first days or even weeks, your head and chattering mind is the wrong place to be.

Focus on doing.

If Your Life Were to End…

What would be left undone or unsaid?

What regrets would there be?

Would people say,

"Geez, she had so much potential, but she just couldn't get it together?"

Or would they say:

"She had such a full life,"

I Give You Permission.

Your old life has ended.

You are free to start a new one.

You can be Sober Ever After.

Love,

Jackie xx

Summary of Part Three

- Once you are sober, it's important to focus on the rest of your life that can be improved
- Take small steps
- Focus on the small stressors than can turn into bigger problems.
- Create a list
- Divide the list into smaller, do-able tasks – eating the elephant, one bite at a time.
- Don't ignore the less pleasant tasks – do these first.
- Deal with debt – it's often a stress that can lead to drinking.
- Learn how to be "financially sober"
- Over consumption is, in many ways, similar to drinking.
- Sobriety can be a tool for the rest of your life.
- Sober "lessons" can be applied to your career or business
- A spiritual epiphany is not necessary.
- The woo- woo stuff can benefit, but simple things can connect you to your Higher Power.
- Helping others can help you.
- If you have read this book, but not yet started – now is the time!

Enjoy this book? You can make a big difference

Reviews are the most powerful tools I have when it comes to getting attention for my books. Much as I'd like to, I don't have the financial resources of a big publisher to spread my sober message! I can't take out full page ads in the newspaper, or put posters on billboards.

(Not yet, anyway)

But I do have something much more powerful and effective than that.

A committed and loyal bunch of readers

Honest reviews of my books help bring them to the attention of other reader. And who knows? It might just be at the time when someone is struggling, or needs a bit of a boost.

If you have enjoyed this book, and found it helpful, I would be very grateful if you would leave review on the book's Amazon page.

Get a FREE ebook!

Building a relationship with my readers is the very best thing about writing. I send regular newsletters with details of new releases, links to my blogs and podcast episodes and articles.

If you sign up to my mailing list, I'll send you a copy of my ebook "Ten Simple Steps. Get Unstuck and Kick the Booze"

Visit www.iamrunningonsober

Have you Read Sober Ever After?

Jackie Elliott loves her wine. It makes her feel confident and helps to relieve her anxiety. Drinking wine is normal! Drinking wine is fun!

Until it isn't.

Jackie refuses to believe she has problem, after all she doesn't live under a bridge, she is still quite thin (and therefore healthy), and is quite able to function!

As Jackie's "Drunken Magical Thinking" propels her into a toxic relationship, and her life begins to disintegrate, Jackie has this nagging thought that maybe she should cut down on the booze..

When Jackie starts to have blackouts – complete gaps in her memory after only a few glasses of wine, she suspects that the party might be coming to an end.

Is Jackie's love affair with Wine really over forever?

From the lowest moments, to her first stumbling sober steps, Jackie shares her thought provoking, sometimes funny, sometimes sad journey to sobriety.

'Sober Ever After' is a memoir from an award

winning sober blogger who fell for the Big Alcohol Con and believed that life wasn't worth living without her beloved booze.

If you are tired of waking up with a hangover, and have started to wonder if there is more to life than the couch and chardonnay, this book is a must read! Buy Sober Ever After and start your own sober journey today!

Dedication

To my patient husband Bob, who supports me, no matter what, and the Sober Blogging Community.

Jackie Elliott

Jackie lives on Vancouver Island with her husband Bob and Att the Cat. You can find her at her online home at www.iamrunningonsober and follow her on Facebook or Instagram